Handbook of Oral Disease

Handbook of Oral Disease

Diagnosis and Management

Revised edition

Crispian Scully CBE

MD PhD MDS MRCS FDSRCS FDSRCPS FFDRCSI FDSRCSE FRCPath FMedSci

Professor
Dean and Director of Studies and Research
Eastman Dental Institute and Hospital for Oral Health Care Sciences
and International Centres for Excellence in Dentistry
Co-Director, World Health Organization Collaborating Centre for
Oral Health, Disability and Culture, University of London
Honorary Consultant at University College London Hospitals,
Great Ormond Street Hospital for Children, London,
the John Radcliffe Hospital, Oxford and the
European Institute for Oncology, Milan

Martin Dunitz

© Martin Dunitz 1999, revised edition 2001

First published in the United Kingdom in 1999 by
Martin Dunitz Ltd
The Livery House
7–9 Pratt Street
London NW1 0AE
Tel. (44) 20 7482 2202

A CIP catalogue record for this title is available from the British Library

ISBN 1-84184-087-4

Distributed in the United States and Canada by:
Thieme New York
333 Seventh Avenue
New York, NY 10001
USA
Tel. 212 760 0888, ext 110

Publisher's note

This book includes photographs that predate the recommendations on
control of cross-infection: gloves should be worn where appropriate.

Composition by Scribe Design, Gillingham, Kent
Printed and bound in Singapore by Kyodo Printing Co (S'pore) Pte Ltd

Contents

To Frances and Zoe

Preface to first edition

An increasingly aging population, advances in medical and surgical sciences, and lifestyle changes that have led to the advent of diseases such as infection with the human immunodeficiency virus (HIV) have resulted in a changing pattern of orofacial diseases. The importance of the prevention and management of orofacial diseases has thus been highlighted. The realization that oral health is important in patients with systemic disorders is growing, and the role of dental staff as oral physicians is increasingly promoted.

This book is intended to be used by all members of the dental team who need a ready office reference. It covers the more common and important soft tissue orofacial disorders and gives clinically relevant aspects of the aetiology, diagnosis, treatment and, where possible, the prevention. Several rare and exotic diseases are also mentioned, since these are seen increasingly worldwide. For greater detail, explanation of rarer disorders and references the reader is referred to Scully C, Flint S, Porter S, *Oral Diseases*, 2nd edn (Martin Dunitz: London, 1996) and Scully C, Cawson RA, *Medical Problems in Dentistry*, 4th edn (Wright: Oxford, 1998).

The disorders have been presented alphabetically to aid easy reference. Patients present with symptoms and/or signs; the first part of the book therefore deals with the symptoms and signs of orofacial disease. Disorders are subsequently described by the main sites affected.

Most conditions are discussed systematically, starting with a definition and then noting the prevalence as *common* (expected to be seen regularly by all practitioners), *uncommon* (seen infrequently), or *rare* (may never be seen). The main age group affected is given as are any clear gender predilections. Clinical features are discussed and illustrations included of the more common conditions. A number of examples are included where the condition is frequently seen but space precludes illustrations of very rare disorders. The essential points of diagnosis and management are summarized.

Principles of diagnosis and management are summarized in a separate chapter. The main drugs in use are tabulated and typical doses for adults provided. Doses should be reduced in children, the elderly and in some medically compromised patients, or those on treatments which might result in interactions. For greater detail on these aspects the reader is referred to Scully C, Epstein J, Wiesenfeld D, *Oxford Handbook of Dental Patient Care* (Oxford University Press: Oxford, 1998). It is always vital to check drug doses, contraindications and adverse effects, and discuss these fully with the patient. Informed consent is required for any treatment.

Dental staff of the future will become much more involved in their roles as oral physicians and thus must regard the patient as a whole. Many of the conditions are rare, but new or unrecognized disorders are appearing all the time. Continued education and access to electronic means of searching the literature are essential. It is also important for all to recognize their limitations; if in doubt, ask.

Finally, I acknowledge my many friends and colleagues in oral medicine and pathology whose advice and help have assisted my understanding of this complex field. I am especially grateful to Stephen Porter, Rod Cawson, John Eveson, Joel Epstein, Oslei Almeida and Stephen Flint, who have helped with illustrative material, some of which was included in *Oral Diseases*.

Further detail can be obtained from Scully C, Almeida OP, Bozzo L et al, *An Atlas of Oral Diagnosis (Atlas De Diagnostico Bucal)*, (Livraria Santos editora: Sao Paulo, 1992); Scully, C, Welbury R, *A Colour Atlas of Oral Diseases in Children and Adolescents* (Mosby Wolfe Medical: London, 1994), and Eveson JW, Scully C, *Colour Atlas of Oral Pathology* (Mosby-Wolfe: London, 1995).

Crispian Scully
London

1

Oral symptoms and signs

Anaesthesia and hypoaesthesia

Normal facial sensation is important to protect the skin, oral mucosa and especially the cornea from damage. Facial sensory awareness may be:

- Completely lost (anaesthesia);
- Partially lost (hypoaesthesia).

Facial sensory loss is caused mainly by extracranial lesions of the trigeminal nerve. Anaesthetic injections (Figure 1.1) or lesions of a sensory branch of the trigeminal nerve may cause anaesthesia or hypoaesthesia in the distribution of the affected branch. Facial sensory loss may lead to corneal, facial or oral ulceration (Figure 1.2). The term paraesthesia does not mean loss of sensation; it means abnormal sensation.

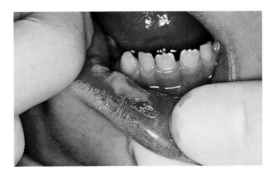

Figure 1.1
Lip ulceration after local analgesic injection in a child who has unwittingly bitten the lip

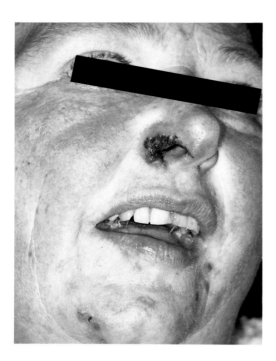

Figure 1.2
*Facial damage after
sensory loss in lesion
affecting trigeminal
nerve*

Extracranial causes of sensory loss

Extracranial causes of facial sensory loss include damage to the trigeminal nerve mainly from the following:

- Trauma;
- Osteomyelitis;
- Malignant disease.

Trauma to a branch of the trigeminal nerve is the usual cause. The mandibular division or its nerve branches may be traumatized by inferior alveolar local analgesic injections, fractures or surgery (particularly osteotomies or surgical extraction of lower third molars), rarely by osteomyelitis or tumour deposits. The lingual nerve may be damaged, especially during removal of lower third molars, particularly when the lingual split technique is used. Occasionally the mental foramen is close beneath a lower denture and there is anaesthesia of the lower lip on the affected side as a result of pressure from the denture. Labial anaesthesia or hypoaesthesia may follow lip surgery, labial gland biopsy or removal of a mucocele.

Osteomyelitis in the mandible may affect the inferior alveolar nerve to cause lower labial anaesthesia. Malignant disease in the mandible or pterygomandibular space may cause lower labial anaesthesia. This may include metastases, leukaemias or gammopathies. Nasopharyngeal carcinomas may invade the pharyngeal wall to infiltrate the mandibular division of the trigeminal nerve, causing pain and sensory loss and, by occluding the Eustachian tube, deafness (Trotter's syndrome).

Damage to branches of the maxillary division of the trigeminal may be caused by trauma (middle-third facial or zygomatic fractures) or a tumour such as carcinoma of the antrum.

Intracranial causes of sensory loss

Serious intracranial causes of sensory loss are uncommon but include the following:

- Multiple sclerosis;
- Brain tumours;
- Syringobulbia;
- Sarcoidosis;
- Infections (e.g. HIV);
- Others (see below).

Since other cranial nerves are anatomically close, there may be associated neurological deficits. In posterior fossa lesions for example, there may be cerebellar features such as ataxia. In middle cranial fossa lesions, there may be associated neurological deficits affecting cranial nerve VI. Less defined causes include:

- **Benign trigeminal neuropathy** is a transient sensory loss of unknown aetiology, in one or more divisions of the trigeminal nerve. The neuropathy seldom appears until the second decade and fortunately the corneal reflex is retained.
- **Psychogenic causes** such as hysteria, and hyperventilation syndrome, may underlie some causes of facial anaesthesia.
- **Organic causes** include conditions such as diabetes or connective tissue disorders.
- **Ritonavir**, other HIV protease inhibitors, and some other drugs can cause circumoral paraesthesia.

Diagnosis

In view of the potential seriousness of facial sensory loss, a full neurological assessment must be undertaken. It is important in patients complaining of facial sensory loss to test all areas, but particularly the corneal reflex. Lesions involving the ophthalmic division of the trigeminal cause corneal anaesthesia, which is tested by gently touching the cornea with a wisp of cotton wool twisted to a point. Normally, this procedure causes a blink but, if the cornea is anaesthetic (or if there is facial palsy), no blink follows, provided that the patient does not actually see the cotton wool. Progressive lesions affecting the sensory part of the trigeminal nerve initially result in a diminishing response to pin-prick of the skin and then complete anaesthesia. Later there may be corneal, facial or oral ulceration (Figure 1.2). Since, in the case of posterior or middle cranial fossa lesions, other cranial nerves are anatomically close, there may be associated neurological deficits. Computerised tomography (CT) or magnetic resonance imaging (MRI) may be indicated to exclude or define organic disorders.

If the patient complains of complete facial or hemifacial anaesthesia, but the corneal reflex is retained or there is apparent anaesthesia over the angle of the mandible (an area not innervated by the trigeminal nerve), then the symptoms are probably functional (nonorganic).

Management

If the cornea is anaesthetic, a protective eye pad should be worn and a tarsorrhaphy (an operation to unite the upper and lower eyelids) may be indicated, since the protective corneal reflex is lost and the cornea may be traumatized.

Dry mouth (xerostomia)

Dry mouth (Figure 1.3) is a frequent, and the most common, salivary complaint but is not always confirmed by evidence of xerostomia. Saliva is essential to oral health, and patients who lack salivary flow suffer from lack of oral lubrication, affecting many functions, and may develop infections as a consequence of the reduced defences.

Anxiety is the most common cause of a dry mouth. The main other causes of dry mouth are iatrogenic; there is no doubt that drugs are the most common cause (Table 1.1), particularly those with anticholinergic or sympathomimetic activity. Irradiation of the salivary glands, cytotoxic chemotherapy and graft-versus-host disease are less common iatrogenic causes.

Disease of glands such as Sjögren's syndrome, sarcoidosis or HIV disease also cause xerostomia. Dehydration, as in diabetes, is an occasional cause. Rarely is there salivary gland agenesis.

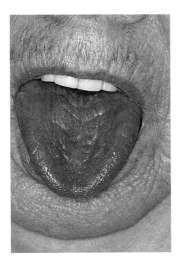

Figure 1.3
Dry mouth in Sjögren's syndrome

Table 1.1   Causes of dry mouth

Iatrogenic
    Drugs
        Anticholinergic drugs such as tricyclics, phenothiazines and
           antihistamines
        Sympathomimetic drugs such as some antihypertensive agents
        Cytotoxic drugs
        Retinoids
        Others such as lithium, opioids, protease inhibitors or didanosine
    Irradiation
    Graft versus host disease
Disease
    Dehydration
    Psychogenic
    Salivary gland disease
        Salivary aplasia
        Sjögren's syndrome
        Sarcoidosis
        HIV salivary gland disease
        Hepatitis C infection

Clinical features

There may be:

- Difficulty in eating dry foods such as biscuits (the cracker sign); controlling dentures in speech and swallowing; and speaking, as the tongue tends to stick to the palate;

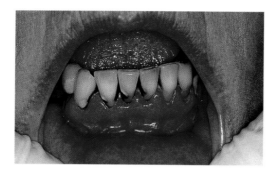

Figure 1.4
Caries in xerostomia

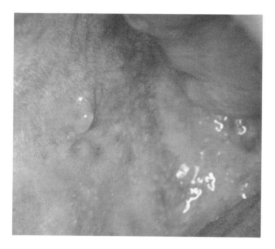

Figure 1.5
Sialadenitis in xerostomia: pus exuding from the parotid duct

- Soreness;
- Unpleasant taste or loss of sense of taste.

Complications may include:

- Dental caries which tend to be severe and difficult to control (Figure 1.4);
- Candidiasis;
- Ascending (suppurative) sialadenitis (Figure 1.5).

Diagnosis

This is a clinical diagnosis mainly. In true xerostomia, the dry mucosa may become tacky and the lips adhere one to another. Lipstick may be seen sticking to the teeth. There may be a lack of salivary pooling in the floor of the mouth, or the saliva may appear scanty or frothy. Saliva may not be expressible from the parotid duct. An examining dental mirror may often stick to the mucosa.

Other investigations may be indicated, including serology and other tests for systemic disease, and salivary function studies, which include the following:

Salivary flow rates (sialometry)

Salivary flow rate estimation is a sensitive indicator of salivary gland dysfunction but is nonspecific. It is carried out by allowing the patient to dribble into a measuring container over 15 minutes; a normal flow exceeds 1.5 ml/15 min.

Salivary biopsy

As biopsy of a parotid gland can result in damage to the facial nerve, a salivary fistula and/or scarring, biopsy of minor salivary glands is usually done. The glands selected are those in the lower labial mucosa (labial gland biopsy), since they are simply biopsied through an incision inside the labial mucosa (Figure 1.6) with few adverse effects except occasional minor hypoaesthesia.

Sialography

Sialography, in which radiopaque dye is introduced into the salivary duct, may be of value if there is duct obstruction or dilatation (Figure 1.7) but carries the risks of discomfort and infection.

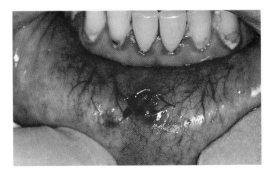

Figure 1.6
Labial salivary gland biopsy

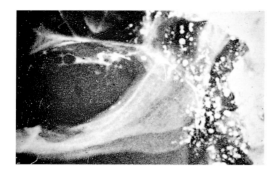

Figure 1.7
Sialography

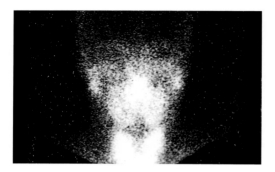

Figure 1.8
Scintiscanning

Salivary scintiscanning

Salivary scintiscanning with technetium pertechnetate correlates both with salivary flow rate and labial gland histopathological changes, and offers the additional advantage that all major salivary glands are examined noninvasively, simultaneously and, if necessary, continuously (Figure 1.8). However, it is not always available, and is expensive and associated with a small radiation hazard.

Ultrasound

Ultrasound, if available, is useful mainly where a neoplasm is suspected.

Sialochemistry

Sialochemistry (studies of constituents of saliva) is of only limited clinical value.

However, in patients complaining of a dry mouth, xerostomia cannot always be objectively confirmed. There is *not* always reduced salivary flow or a salivary disorder. There may be a psychogenic reason for the complaint.

Management

Any underlying cause of xerostomia should if possible be rectified. The lips may need protection with petroleum jelly. It is also wise for the patient to avoid dry foods such as biscuits, and anything that may produce xerostomia, such as:

- Drugs (for example tricyclic antidepressants);
- Alcohol;
- Smoking.

Salivation may be stimulated by using:

- Chewing gums (containing sorbitol, not sucrose);
- Diabetic sweets;
- Cholinergic drugs that stimulate salivation (sialogogues), such as pilocarpine (Table 10.11). These drugs should be used by the specialist since unfortunately they may cause other cholinergic effects such as bradycardia, sweating and the urge to urinate. Pyridostigmine is of greater benefit since it is longer acting and associated with fewer adverse effects.

Salivary substitutes may help symptomatically. Various substitutes are available (Chapter 10) including water, methylcellulose and mucin. Salivary substitutes usually contain carboxymethylcellulose (Glandosane, Luborant, Salivace, Saliveze) or mucin (Saliva Orthana). Glandosane is effective but has a lowish pH and may thus not be suitable. Saliva Orthana contains fluoride (Table 10.11).

Dental caries

Dietary control of sucrose intake, and the daily use of fluorides (1% sodium fluoride gels or 0.4% stannous fluoride gels) are essential to control dental caries. Regular dental checks are required.

Candidiasis

Dentures should be left out of the mouth at night and stored in sodium hypochlorite solution or chlorhexidine. An antifungal such as miconazole gel or amphotericin or nystatin ointment should be spread on the denture before reinsertion and a topical antifungal preparation such as nystatin, amphotericin suspension or lozenges used. Fluconazole is also effective.

Bacterial sialadenitis

Acute sialadenitis needs treating with a penicillinase-resistant antibiotic such as flucloxacillin.

Halitosis

Halitosis, or oral malodour, is a fairly common complaint in adults. It is common on awakening (morning breath) and then often has no special significance. With halitosis from any cause, the patient may also complain of a bad taste (page 28).

Oral sepsis is the most usual cause of halitosis, but smoking and eating various foods are also well-known causes. Sepsis in the respiratory tract may occasionally be causal, as can other systemic diseases such as diabetes. The following are the main causes:

- Periodontal sepsis (Figure 1.9);
- Other types of oral sepsis;
- Infected extraction sockets are also likely to contain anaerobic infections and give rise to halitosis.

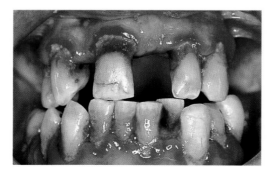

Figure 1.9
Periodontal disease: a common cause of halitosis

- Food packing or a neglected or poorly designed dental bridge or appliance;
- Ulcers;
- Dry mouth;
- Starvation;
- Smoking;
- Some foods (e.g. garlic, durian, curries, onions);
- Drugs (e.g. alcohol, solvent abuse, chloral hydrate, nitrites and nitrates, dimethyl sulphoxide, cytotoxic drugs);
- Diabetic ketosis: the breath may smell of acetone;
- Nasal sepsis or foreign bodies, or infection of the paranasal sinuses or lower respiratory tract;
- Gastrointestinal disease;
- Hepatic failure;
- Renal failure;
- Psychogenic factors. The complaint of halitosis may be made by patients who do not have it but imagine it because of psychogenic disorders.

Diagnosis

- Assessment of halitosis is usually subjective;
- A few centres have the apparatus (Halimeter) for objectively measuring the responsible volatile sulphur compounds (methyl mercaptan, hydrogen sulphide, dimethyl sulphide);
- Microbiological investigations such as the BANA (benzoyl arginine naphthylamide) test can be helpful.

Management

The management includes:

- Treatment of the cause;
- Regular meals;
- Abstinence from smoking and foods such as onions and garlic;
- Improving oral hygiene—prophylaxis, toothbrushing, flossing, chlorhexidine, cetylpyridinium or other mouthwashes (Table 10.1);
- Chewing gum;
- Using proprietary 'fresh breath' sprays, lozenges, mouthwashes, or other preparations;
- Brushing or scraping the tongue.

Hyperpigmentation

The most usual cause of brown oral mucosal pigmentation is ethnic, mainly in Blacks, but may be seen even in some fairly light-skinned people. It is most obvious in the anterior labial gingivae (Figure 1.10). Causes of hyperpigmentation are shown in Table 1.2.

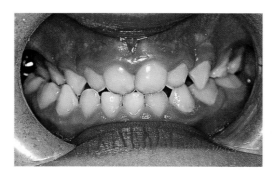

Figure 1.10
Racial pigmentation in a child

Table 1.2   Causes of hyperpigmentation

Localized	Amalgam, graphite or other tattoos, ephelis (freckle), naevus, melanotic macules, melanoacanthoma, malignant melanoma, Kaposi's sarcoma, epithelioid angiomatosis, verruciform xanthoma
Multiple or generalized	
Genetic	Race, Peutz–Jegher's syndrome, Laugier–Hunziker syndrome, complex of myxomas, spotty pigmentation and endocrine overactivity, Carney syndrome, Leopard syndrome, lentiginosis profusa
Drugs	Smoking, betel, antimalarials, amiodarone, minocycline, chlorpromazine, ACTH, zidovudine, clofazimine, ketoconazole, methyldopa, busulphan, menthol, contraceptive pill, metals
Endocrine	Addison's disease, Albright's syndrome, pregnancy
Postinflammatory	Especially seen in lichen planus
Others	Haemochromatosis, Albright's syndrome, generalized neurofibromatosis, incontinentia pigmenti, Whipple's disease, Wilson's disease, Gaucher's disease, HIV disease, thalassaemia

Diagnosis

The nature of hyperpigmentation can sometimes only be established after further investigation. In particular, for generalized or multiple hyperpigmentation:

* Blood pressure should be taken to exclude the hypotension of Addison's disease;
* Blood tests may be needed if Addison's disease is suspected; plasma cortisol levels and a Synacthen test may be indicated.

For localized hyperpigmentation:

* Radiographs may be helpful whenever hyperpigmentation may be caused by amalgam, graphite or a foreign body;
* Photographs may be useful for future comparison;
* A biopsy may be indicated.

Management

Management is of the underlying condition.

Loss of elasticity of oral tissues

Scarring or loss of elasticity may be seen in the following:

* Burns (from heat, cold, chemicals, electricity or irradiation);
* Oral submucous fibrosis;
* Scleroderma;
* Epidermolysis bullosa;
* Pemphigoid and some other inflammatory conditions.

Lumps and swellings

Patients often notice a lump first because it becomes sore. It is not unknown for individuals to discover and worry about anatomical lumps. Pathological causes of lumps and swellings include a range of different conditions (Table 1.3).

Table 1.3   Conditions which may present as lumps or swellings in the mouth

Normal	Pterygoid hamulus, parotid papillae, foliate or circumvallate papillae, unerupted teeth
Developmental	Haemangioma, lymphangioma, maxillary and mandibular tori, hereditary gingival fibromatosis, von Recklinghausen's neurofibromatosis
Inflammatory	Abscess, pyogenic granuloma, Crohn's disease, orofacial granulomatosis, sarcoidosis, Wegener's granulomatosis, others
Traumatic	Epulis, fibroepithelial polyp, denture granulomata
Cystic	Eruption cysts, developmental cysts, cysts of infective origin
Fibro-osseous	Cherubism, fibrous dysplasia, Paget's disease
Hormonal	Pregnancy epulis/gingivitis, oral contraceptive pill gingivitis
Drugs	Phenytoin, cyclosporin, calcium channel blockers
Blood dyscrasias	Leukaemia and lymphoma
Neoplasms	Benign and malignant
Others	Angioedema, amyloidosis
Multiple lumps	Papillomas, condylomas, papillary hyperplasia, proliferative verrucous leukoplakia, Cowden's syndrome, focal dermal hypoplasia, multiple endocrinopathy syndrome, drug-induced gingival hyperplasia, hereditary gingival fibromatosis, Crohn's disease, orofacial granulomatosis, sarcoidosis

Diagnosis

Apart from the history and location, features of a swelling which can help in reaching the diagnosis include:

- Alteration in size or colour;
- Any discharge from the lesion (clear fluid, pus, blood);
- Duration;
- Pain or tenderness.

The relevant medical history should be fully reviewed, as several systemic disorders may be associated with intraoral or facial swellings. Inspection should include a careful note of the following.

- The location of the lump in relation to anatomical structures present. For example, many midline lesions tend to be developmental in origin (e.g. torus palatinus);
- Whether a lesion is bilateral—few neoplastic lumps are bilateral;

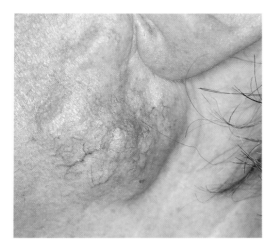

Figure 1.11
*Malignant salivary
neoplasm: the prominent
blood vessels suggest
malignancy*

- The site, shape and size (in millimetres);
- The colour of the lump. A pale-coloured lump may suggest underlying fibrosis or soft tissues stretched over bony enlargement; red suggests inflammation, haemangioma or giant-cell epulis. Any variations in colour within the lump (e.g. the yellow appearance of a 'pointing' abscess) should be observed;
- The surface characteristics. Papillomas have an obvious anemone-like appearance; carcinomas and other malignant lesions and deep mycoses tend to have a nodular surface and often ulcerate;
- Abnormal blood vessels, which suggest a neoplasm (Figures 1.11 and 8.2);
- Whether the swelling has an orifice or sinus. If fluid is draining, see whether it is clear, cloudy or purulent;
- Similar or relevant changes elsewhere in the oral cavity.

Palpation may then help determine whether the lump:

- Contains fluid (fluctuant because of cyst fluid, mucus, pus or blood);
- Is soft, firm or hard like a carcinoma (indurated);
- Is painful (suggesting an inflammatory lesion);
- Releases fluid (e.g. pus from an abscess);
- Blanches (vascular);
- Crackles (like an egg-shell being broken), suggesting a cyst;
- Overlies an underlying structure (e.g. the crown of a tooth under an eruption cyst);
- Is in deeper structures (e.g. submandibular calculus).

Bimanual palpation should be used when investigating lesions in the submandibular salivary glands, floor of the mouth, cheek and occasionally the tongue.

Investigations

The nature of many lumps can only be established after further investigation. In particular:

- Any teeth adjacent to a lump in the jaw should be tested for vitality, and any caries or suspect restorations should be investigated;
- The periodontal status of any involved teeth should be determined;
- Radiographs are required whenever lumps involve the jaws, and should show the full extent of the lesion and possibly other areas. Special radiographs (e.g. of the skull, sinuses, salivary gland function), CT scans or MRI or other investigations may, on occasions, be indicated;
- Photographs may be useful for future comparison;
- Blood tests may be needed if there is suspicion of a blood dyscrasia or endocrinopathy. Special blood tests (e.g. for autoantibodies) may be indicated for suspected vesiculobullous lesions;
- Biopsy may be indicated.

Management

Management is of the underlying condition.

Pain

A wide range of conditions can be responsible for pain (Table 1.4).
Local odontogenic cause (Figure 1.12).
Temporomandibular pain dysfunction (Chapter 3).
Paranasal sinus and nasopharynx disease. In acute sinusitis:

- There has usually been a preceding cold followed by local pain and tenderness (but not swelling);
- There is radio-opacity of the affected sinuses, sometimes with an obvious fluid level;
- Pain may be aggravated by change of position of the head. With maxillary sinusitis, pain may be felt in related upper molars,

Table 1.4   Causes of orofacial pain

Local disorders	Oral, ENT
Referred pain	Nasopharyngeal, ocular, aural, cardiorespiratory
Neurological disorders	Idiopathic trigeminal neuralgia, malignant neoplasms involving the trigeminal nerve, glossopharyngeal neuralgia, herpes zoster (including postherpetic neuralgia)
Vascular disorders	Migraine, migrainous neuralgia, giant-cell arteritis
Psychogenic causes	Atypical facial pain, burning mouth syndrome, temporomandibular pain-dysfunction

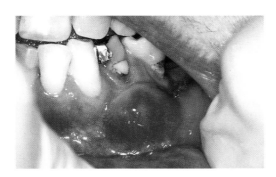

Figure 1.12
Dental abscess causing pain and swelling

which may be tender to percussion. The pain of ethmoidal or sphenoidal sinusitis is deep in the root of the nose;

- Tumours in the sinuses can also cause orofacial pain by infiltrating branches of the trigeminal nerve.

Salivary gland disorders. In children, the most common cause of salivary pain is mumps. In adults, pain from salivary glands results usually from blockage of a salivary duct by calculus or mucus plug. This pain:

- Is localized;
- May be quite severe;
- May be intensified by increased saliva production such as before and with meals.

The affected gland may be swollen and tender to palpation. Mouth-opening may aggravate the pain, and thus there may be some trismus.
Referred pain from:

- Eyes: disorders of refraction, retrobulbar neuritis or glaucoma can cause pain which may radiate to the orbit or frontal region;
- Ears: middle ear disease may cause headaches;

- Neck: neck pain, usually from cervical spondylosis, occasionally causes pain referred to the face;
- Chest: Cardiac pain (angina) and lung cancer pain can be referred to the jaws.

Neurological causes. Idiopathic trigeminal neuralgia is an important cause of pain, but similar severe orofacial pain can result from cerebrovascular disease, multiple sclerosis, infections such as HIV infection, or neoplasms. Physical signs such as facial sensory or motor impairment may then be present.

Vascular causes. Migraine, migrainous neuralgia and cranial arteritis may cause orofacial pain.

Psychogenic disorders. There is a range of types of orofacial pain for which no organic cause can be identified even with sophisticated techniques, and which appear to have a psychogenic basis. It must be stressed that such a diagnosis should be made only where there has been very careful exclusion of organic disease.

Psychogenic orofacial pain can be seen in:

- Normal persons under stress;
- Persons with a personality trait, such as hypochondriasis;
- Neurotic, often depressed persons;
- Psychotic or mentally challenged patients.

Features common to these types of psychogenic pain are as follows:

- They are chronic, often of a constant dull boring or burning type;
- Location may be ill-defined;
- Symptoms do not waken the patient from sleep;
- Objective signs and all investigations are negative;
- The patient often appears otherwise quite well;
- Adverse life-events, such as bereavement or family illness may precede the onset;
- Multiple oral and/or other psychogenic-related complaints, such as headaches, chronic back pains, irritable bowel syndrome or dysmenorrhoea are common;
- Few patients seem to try or persist in using analgesics;
- Many patients are middle-aged or older females;
- Multiple consultations are common;
- Some patients respond to antidepressants such as dothiepin, but others refuse psychiatric help or medication;
- Cure is uncommon.

Management

Management is of the underlying condition, and use of analgesics (Table 10.3).

Paralysis

The common causes of facial paralysis are:

- Strokes (upper motor neurone lesions), seen mainly in older males;
- Bell's palsy (lower motor neurone lesions) seen mainly in younger patients.

Occasionally, a temporary facial palsy follows the administration of an inferior alveolar local analgesic if the anaesthetic solution tracks through the parotid gland to reach the facial nerve (Figure 1.13). Other causes are shown in Table 1.5. The neurones to the upper face receive

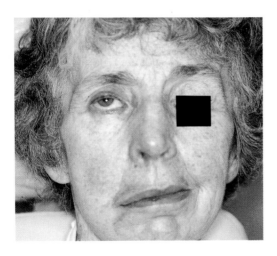

Figure 1.13
Facial palsy after misplaced local analgesic injection. The right inferior alveolar injection entered the parotid gland and thus anaesthetized the facial nerve within the gland

Table 1.5   Causes of facial palsy

Upper motor neurone lesion	Cerebrovascular accident, trauma, tumour, infection, multiple sclerosis
Lower motor neurone lesion	
Systemic infection	Bell's palsy (herpes simplex virus usually), Varicella-Zoster virus infection, Lyme disease, HIV infection
Middle ear disease	Otitis media, cholesteatoma
Lesion of skull base	Fracture, infection
Parotid lesion	Tumour
Trauma to branch of facial nerve	

Table 1.6   Differentiation of upper (UMN) from lower motor neurone (LMN) lesions of the facial nerve

	LMN lesions	*UMN lesions*
Emotional movements of face	Lost	Retained
Blink reflex	Lost	Retained
Ability to wrinkle forehead	Lost	Retained
Drooling from commissure	Common	Uncommon
Lacrimation, taste or hearing	May be affected	Unaffected

bilateral upper motor neurone (UMN) innervation. Upper motor neurone facial palsy is usually caused by damage in the middle capsule of the brain. Damage thus extends to other areas, including motor neurones, but extrapyramidal influences can still act on the face, for example, on laughing, because of the bilateral cortical representation. An UMN lesion, therefore, is characterized by unilateral facial palsy, with some sparing of the frontalis and orbicularis oculi muscles; the face may still move with emotional responses (because of extrapyramidal influences) and there may also be a paresis of the ipsilateral arm or arm and leg, or some aphasia.

In contrast, lower motor neurone (LMN) facial palsy is characterized by total unilateral paralysis of all muscles of facial expression, both for voluntary and emotional responses, but no hemiparesis, since the facial nerve neurones supplying the lower face receive upper motor neurones only for the contralateral motor cortex. Features that differentiate UMN lesions from LMN lesions are outlined in Table 1.6.

Diagnosis

In facial palsy:

- Facial weakness is demonstrated by asking the patient to close the eyes against resistance, raise the eyebrows, raise the lips to show the teeth (Figure 1.14), and try to whistle;
- The forehead is unfurrowed;
- The patient is unable to close the eye on that side;
- The eye rolls upwards (Bell's sign) on attempted closure;
- Tears tend to overflow onto the cheek (epiphora);
- The nasolabial fold is obliterated;
- The corner of the mouth droops.

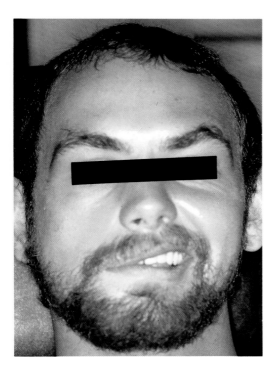

Figure 1.14
Right-sided Bell's palsy: the patient is attempting to smile

The following investigations are indicated:

- Full neurological examination, looking particularly for signs suggesting a central lesion, such as hemiparesis, tremor, loss of balance, or involvement of the Vth, VIth or VIIIth cranial nerves;
- Test for loss of hearing;
- Test for taste loss;
- Aural examination for discharge and other signs of middle ear disease;
- Blood pressure measurement (to exclude hypertension);
- Fasting blood sugar levels (to exclude diabetes);
- In some areas, Lyme disease (tick-borne infection with *Borrelia burgdorferi*) should be excluded by serology;
- HIV infection may need to be considered.

Management

Management is of the underlying condition.

Purpura

Purpura is bleeding into the skin and mucosa, usually caused by trauma, suction or a blood platelet disorder (Table 1.7). Occasional small traumatic petechiae at the occlusal line are seen in otherwise healthy patients. Localized oral purpura or angina bullosa haemorrhagica is another fairly common cause seen mainly in the soft palate, in older persons (Chapter 8). Red or brown pinpoint lesions (petechiae) or diffuse bruising (ecchymoses) are seen, mainly at sites of trauma, such as at the junction of the hard and soft palate (Figure 1.15).

Table 1.7   Causes of oral purpura

Trauma	Suction or trauma from appliances, habits, fellatio, cunnilingus, vomiting
Platelet disorders	
Autoimmune	(ITP; idiopathic thrombocytopenic purpura)
Bone marrow disorders	Aplastic anaemia, leukaemia
Infections	Infectious mononucleosis, rubella, HIV infection
Gammopathies	
Rare disorders	Chediak–Higashi syndrome, Wiskott–Aldrich syndrome, Fanconi's anaemia, Glanzmann's disease, Moschcowitz disease (thrombotic thrombocytopenia), Henoch–Schönlein purpura
Localized oral purpura (angina bullosa haemorrhagica)	
Vascular disorders	Scurvy
Amyloidosis	

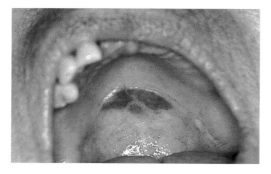

Figure 1.15
Palatal purpura at a typical site of trauma

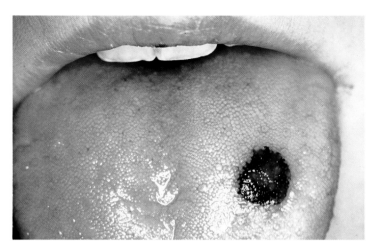

Figure 1.16
Purpura on the tongue

Diagnosis

The diagnosis is mainly clinical (Figure 1.16). Lesions may be seen on the skin or other mucosae, and they do not blanch on pressure (cf. haemangioma). It may be necessary to take a blood picture (including blood and platelet count) and assess haemostatic function.

Management

Treatment is of the underlying cause.

Red and bluish lesions

Most red lesions are inflammatory in origin (Figure 1.17). However, it is important to appreciate that others are associated with mucosal atrophy; erythroplasia is one of the more important causing a localized lesion, since it is often dysplastic. Other causes of red lesions are shown in Table 1.8.

Diagnosis

Diagnosis is mainly clinical but haematological tests to exclude vitamin deficiencies, microbiological investigations or biopsy may be indicated.

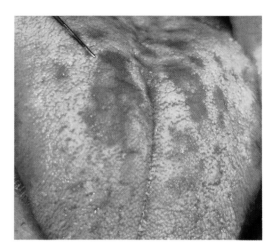

Figure 1.17
*Red lesions due to
erythematous candidiasis*

Table 1.8   Causes of red lesions

Localized	Candidiasis, geographic tongue, lichen planus, lupus erythematosus, erythroplasia, Reiter's disease, purpura, graft-versus-host disease, telangiectases (HHT or scleroderma), angiokeratomas (Fabry's disease), angiomas, Kaposi's sarcoma, epithelioid angiomatosis, burns, avitaminosis B_{12}, drugs
Generalized	Candidiasis, avitaminosis B complex (rarely), irradiation or chemotherapy-induced mucositis, mucosal atrophy, polycythaemia

Management

Treatment is of the underlying cause.

Salivary swellings (see also Chapter 5)

The causes of swelling of the salivary glands are summarized in Table 1.9. Most swellings are caused by salivary duct obstruction (Figure 5.1), but sialadenitis, Sjögren's syndrome, sialosis, sarcoidosis, HIV infection and neoplasms are important causes to be excluded.

Diagnosis

It can be difficult to establish whether a salivary gland is genuinely swollen, especially in obese patients (Figure 1.18). A useful guide to whether the patient is simply obese or has parotid enlargement is to observe the outward deflection of the ear lobe which is seen in true parotid swelling (Figure 1.19). Diagnosis of the cause is mainly clinical but investigations such as serology for autoantibodies or HIV antibodies, liver function tests, or needle or open biopsy may be indicated.

Table 1.9   Causes of salivary gland swelling

Inflammatory	Mumps, ascending sialadenitis, recurrent parotitis, HIV parotitis, other infections (e.g. hepatitis C, tuberculosis), Sjögren's syndrome, sarcoidosis
Cystic fibrosis	
Neoplasms	
Duct obstruction	e.g. sialolithiasis
Sialosis	
Drugs	e.g. phenylbutazone, chlorhexidine
Deposits	e.g. amyloid

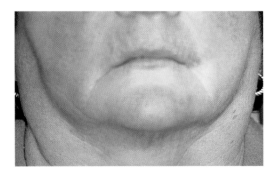

Figure 1.18
Salivary gland swelling

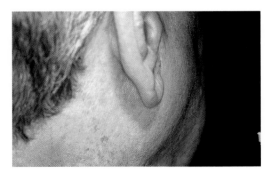

Figure 1.19
Parotid swelling, deflecting ear lobe

Unilateral salivary gland swelling in a child may be caused by:

- Mumps;
- Chronic recurrent parotitis;
- Benign mesenchymal tumours (e.g. haemangioma, fibrous histio-
cytoma, xanthogranuloma).

Bilateral swelling is mainly seen in:

- Mumps;
- HIV salivary gland disease;
- Sialosis;
- Sjögren's syndrome;
- Warthin's tumour.

Management

Treatment is of the underlying cause.

Sialorrhoea (ptyalism)

Infants frequently drool; this is normal, especially when 'teething.'
The complaint of sialorrhoea (excess salivation) at other ages is very
uncommon and not always associated with a genuine increase in saliva production. Causes are shown in Table 1.10.

Table 1.10   Causes of sialorrhoea

Painful oral lesions	
Foreign bodies in the mouth	
Drugs	Anticholinesterases, clozapine, cocaine, iodides, bromides, ammonium bicarbonate, ethyl chloride, dimercaprol, ketamine, ethionamide, digitalis, benzodiazepines
Poor neuromuscular coordination	Cerebral palsy, Parkinson's disease, facial palsy, learning disability, other physical disability
Psychogenic	
Episodic idiopathic paroxysmal sialorrhoea	

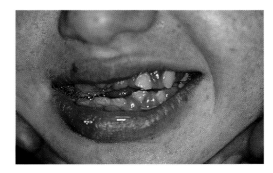

Figure 1.20
*Drooling in learning
disability*

In some cases the complaint relates not to excess saliva production but to an inability to swallow saliva as a result of muscular incoordination, neurological disorders such as Parkinson's disease, cerebral palsy or learning disability, pharyngeal obstruction, or reduced swallowing rate (Figure 1.20).

Diagnosis

Diagnosis is clinical; estimation of salivary flow may be indicated.

Management

- Treatment is of the underlying cause;
- Propantheline bromide 15 mg, or transdermal scopolamine (hyoscine) using dermal patches, may be effective. Other atropinics, though theoretically useful for controlling sialorrhoea, are rarely of practical value because of side-effects;
- Antihistamines are sometimes useful;
- Surgical operations have been devised to reroute the submandibular gland duct to open posteriorly;
- Botulinum toxoid may help;
- Tympanic neurectomy is a last resort.

Staining

Superficial brown discoloration of the teeth and soft tissues—often the dorsum of the tongue—may be caused by:

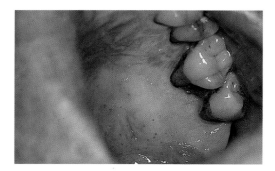

Figure 1.21
Nicotine-staining of teeth

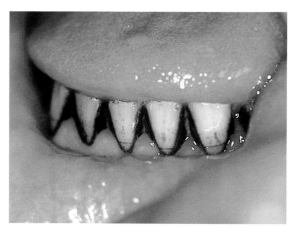

Figure 1.22
Iron staining of teeth

- Tobacco (Figure 1.21);
- Betel;
- Drugs (such as iron salts or griseofulvin) (Figure 1.22);
- Foods and beverages (such as coffee and tea);
- Chlorhexidine;
- Amoxicillin.

Such discoloration is easily removed professionally and is of little consequence. Minocycline stains bone, and may give a blackish colour to the overlying gingiva or mucosa.

Taste disturbances

Taste is susceptible to genetic and hormonal factors. For example, sensitivity to the bitter taste of phenylthiourea is genetically determined.

Taste is susceptible to the general sensory phenomenon known as adaptation, that is the progressive reduction in the appreciation of a stimulus during the course of continual exposure to that stimulus, and can be distorted by various factors. Dry mouth for any reason can distort taste, as can drugs (particularly penicillamine, protease inhibitors and captopril), nutritional deficiencies (especially of zinc), aging and various disorders.

Taste also varies through the menstrual cycle and may be distorted during pregnancy, often with the appearance of cravings for unusual foods.

Causes of *cacogeusia* (an unpleasant taste in the mouth) are given in Table 1.11.

Table 1.11   Causes of unpleasant taste

Poor oral hygiene	
Oral sepsis	
Oroantral fistula	
Starvation	
Dry mouth	
Salivary gland disorders	Sjögren's syndrome, irradiation damage, mumps
Psychogenic causes	Depression, anxiety states, psychoses, hypochondriasis
Foods	Garlic, durian, curries, onions
Drugs	Smoking, alcohol, solvent abuse, chloral hydrate, nitrites and nitrates, metronidazole, gold, lithium, dimethyl sulphoxide, cytotoxic drugs, protease inhibitors, penicillamine, captopril
Respiratory tract infections	
Liver failure and cirrhosis	
Renal failure	
Diabetic ketosis	
Gastrointestinal disease	

Management

Treatment is of the underlying cause.

Loss of the sense of taste may be caused by a range of conditions (Table 1.12). Anosmia commonly produces an apparent loss of sense of taste; probably the most common cause of loss of taste is a viral upper respiratory tract infection. Olfaction may also be impaired after head injuries, due to tearing of olfactory fibres, and in aging, some

Table 1.12   Disorders causing decreased sensation of taste

Oral disorders	Xerostomia, sepsis
Various foods	
Smoking	
Old age	
Irradiation or burns	
Zinc and other deficiencies	
Drugs	Cytotoxics, captopril, carbimazole, clofibrate, lincomycin, penicillamine
Disorders affecting cranial nerves	Damage to lingual nerve, chorda tympani or facial nerve, Bell's palsy
Cerebral disorders	Brain tumours
Psychogenic disorders	

endocrine disorders (especially hypothyroidism), Parkinson's disease and some other cerebral disorders.

Ulcers and erosions

The term erosion is often used for superficial breaches of the epithelium that often have a red appearance since there is little damage to the underlying lamina propria. If a breach penetrates the full thickness of the epithelium, however, it typically becomes covered by a fibrinous exudate and then has a yellowish appearance.

The term ulcer is used usually where there is damage to both epithelium and lamina propria, and then a crater forms, sometimes made more obvious clinically by oedema or proliferation causing swelling of the surrounding tissue. Inflammation, if present, also highlights the ulcer, which often then has a yellow or grey floor with a red halo (Figure 1.23).

Most ulcers/erosions are due to local causes such as trauma or burns (Table 1.13). Some are aphthae, or caused by:

* Malignant neoplasms;
* Drugs (such as cytotoxic agents);
* Systemic disease.

Ulcers and erosions can be the final common manifestation of a spectrum of conditions causing epithelial damage ranging from an immunological attack as in pemphigus, pemphigoid or lichen planus,

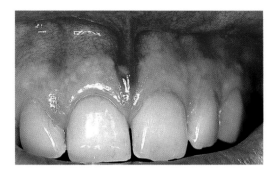

Figure 1.23
Traumatic ulceration of the labial fraenum caused by a toothbrush injury

Table 1.13   Main causes of mouth ulcers

Local causes	Trauma, burns (heat, cold, chemical, radiation, electric)
Recurrent aphthae (and Behçet's syndrome)	
Malignant neoplasms	Oral, or encroaching from antrum
Drugs	Cytotoxics, nicorandil, protease inhibitors, alendronate, many others
Systemic disease	
Microbial disease	Herpetic stomatitis, chickenpox, hand, foot and mouth disease, herpangina, infectious mononucleosis, HIV, acute necrotizing gingivitis, tuberculosis, syphilis, histoplasmosis, cryptococcosis, blastomycosis, paracoccidioidomycosis, leishmaniasis
Mucocutaneous disease	Lichen planus, pemphigus vulgaris, pemphigoid and variants, erythema multiforme, dermatitis herpetiformis, linear IgA disease, epidermolysis bullosa, chronic ulcerative stomatitis, other dermatoses
Blood disorders	Anaemia, immunodeficiencies (leukaemia, myelodysplastic syndrome, primary immunodeficiencies, HIV, neutropenia, other white cell dyscrasias, gammopathies)
Gastrointestinal disease	Coeliac disease, Crohn's disease, ulcerative colitis
Rheumatic diseases	Lupus erythematosus, Behçet's syndrome, Sweet's syndrome
Vasculitides	Wegener's granulomatosis, periarteritis nodosa, giant-cell arteritis
Endocrine	Glucagonoma
Disorders of uncertain pathogenesis	Eosinophilic ulcer, hypereosinophilic syndrome, necrotizing sialometaplasia

to damage resulting from an immune defect as in HIV disease and leukaemia, to infections such as herpesviruses, tuberculosis and syphilis, to nutritional defects as in vitamin deficiencies and those caused by some intestinal diseases.

Ulcers of local causes
These may be seen in:

- Neonates who occasionally develop an ulcer in the palate (Bednar's ulcer). This may be caused by trauma from the examining finger of the paediatrician;
- Children, usually caused by accidental biting, or following dental treatment or other trauma (Figure 1.24), hard foods or appliances (Figure 1.25). In child abuse (nonaccidental injury),

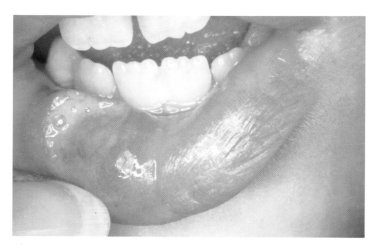

Figure 1.24
Trauma to lip after local analgesic injection

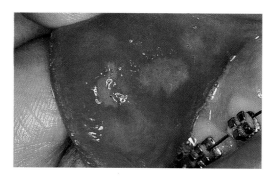

Figure 1.25
Trauma from an orthodontic appliance

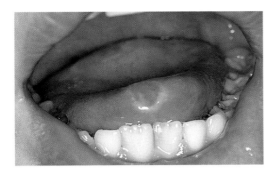

Figure 1.26
Chronic self-induced (artefactual) trauma to the tongue in a mentally challenged patient

ulceration of the upper labial fraenum may follow a traumatic fraenal tear. Bruised and swollen lips, and even subluxed teeth or fractured mandible can be other features of child abuse. The lingual fraenum may be traumatized by repeated rubbing over the lower incisor teeth in children with recurrent bouts of coughing as in whooping cough (termed Riga–Fedes disease). Chronic trauma may produce an ulcer with a keratotic margin (Figure 1.26);

- Adults in whom the lingual fraenum is damaged by trauma in cunnilingus (Figures 1.27–1.29);
- At any age there may be factitious ulceration, especially of the maxillary gingivae (Figures 1.26, 1.30, and 4.174), or burns from chemicals of various kinds, heat, cold or ionizing radiation.

Aphthae. Ulcers are commonly aphthae, usually in persons who are otherwise well. Occasionally they are associated with haematinic deficiencies, or are part of Behçet's syndrome or Periodic Fever, Aphthae, Pharyngitis, and Adenitis (PFAPA) syndrome.

Drugs may induce ulcers by a variety of mechanisms. Cytotoxic drugs are a frequent cause of ulcers.

Neoplasms. A range of neoplasms may present with ulcers; most commonly these are carcinomas, but Kaposi's sarcoma, lymphomas and other neoplasms may be seen.

Systemic disease. Infective causes of mouth ulcers include mainly viruses, especially herpesviruses. Other viruses that may cause mouth ulcers include Coxsackie and ECHO viruses. HIV infection can result in ulcers for a range of reasons, from infections to tumours.

Bacterial causes of mouth ulcers are less common, apart from acute necrotizing ulcerative gingivitis. Syphilis and tuberculosis (TB) are uncommon in the developed world at present.

Fungal causes of ulcers are also uncommon in the developed world but are increasingly seen in immunocompromised persons and travellers. Protozoal causes of ulcers are rare in the developed world.

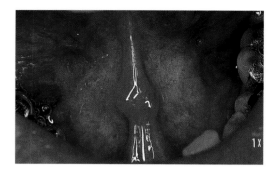

Figure 1.27
Trauma to lingual fraenum from cunnilingus, causing erythema and soreness

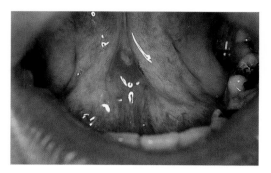

Figure 1.28
Trauma to lingual fraenum from cunnilingus, causing small ulcer

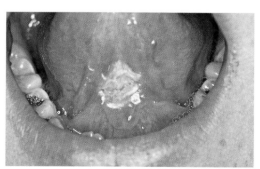

Figure 1.29
Trauma to lingual fraenum from cunnilingus, causing deep ulceration

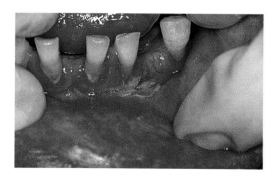

Figure 1.30
Factitious (self-induced) ulceration

Mucocutaneous disorders that may cause oral ulceration include particularly lichen planus, occasionally pemphigoid and rarely pemphigus and erythema multiforme. Lesions resembling pemphigoid, however, may be due to any of a heterogeneous group of autoimmune mucocutaneous disorders including pemphigoid variants, dermatitis herpetiformis and linear IgA disease.

Haematological disease can cause ulcers. Mouth ulcers may be seen in leukaemias, associated with cytotoxic therapy, viral, bacterial or fungal infection, or other nonspecific causes. Other oral features may include purpura, gingival bleeding, recurrent herpes labialis and candidiasis.

Gastrointestinal disorders may result in ulcers. A small number of patients with aphthae have intestinal disease such as coeliac disease causing malabsorption and deficiencies of haematinics, when they may also develop angular stomatitis or glossitis. Orofacial features of Crohn's disease, in addition to mouth ulcers, may include facial and/or labial swelling; angular stomatitis and/or cracked lips; mucosal tags and/or cobble-stoning; or gingival hyperplasia. Pyostomatitis vegetans is a rare complication seen in inflammatory bowel diseases.

Diagnosis

The diagnosis is based on the history and clinical features. General physical examination is indicated unless the cause is undoubtedly local. Investigations are often indicated.

Biopsy may be needed, especially where there

- is a single ulcer persisting more than 3 weeks;
- is induration;
- are skin lesions, lesions in other mucosae, or other related systemic lesions.

Blood tests may be useful for excluding possible deficiencies or other conditions when a systemic cause is suspected.

Chest radiography and other special investigations may be indicated where there are possible pulmonary lesions such as TB, the deep mycoses, carcinoma or sarcoidosis.

Features that might suggest a systemic background to mouth ulcers include the following.

Extraoral features such as:

- Skin lesions;
- Ocular lesions;
- Genital lesions;
- Purpura;
- Fever;

- Lymphadenopathy;
- Hepatomegaly;
- Splenomegaly;
- Chronic cough;
- Gastrointestinal complaints (e.g. pain, altered bowel habits, blood in faeces);
- Loss of weight or, in children, a failure to thrive;
- Weakness.

An atypical history or ulcer behaviour such as:

- Onset of ulcers in later adult life;
- Exacerbation of ulcers;
- Severe aphthae;
- Aphthae unresponsive to topical hydrocortisone or triamcinolone.

Other oral lesions, especially:

- Candidiasis;
- Glossitis;
- Petechiae;
- Gingival bleeding;
- Gingival swelling;
- Necrotizing gingivitis;
- Herpetic lesions;
- Hairy leukoplakia;
- Kaposi's sarcoma.

Management

- Treat the underlying cause.
- Remove aetiological factors.
- Prescribe a chlorhexidine 0.2% aqueous mouthwash (Table 10.1).
- Maintain good oral hygiene.
- A benzydamine mouthwash or spray may help ease discomfort (Table 10.2).

Most ulcers of local cause heal spontaneously in about 1–2 weeks if the cause is removed and such supportive care is given.

White lesions

Lesions appear white usually because they are composed of thickened keratin, which looks white when wet (Figure 1.31). Most are acquired; they are discussed in Chapter 4 (Table 1.14).

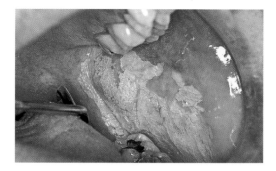

Figure 1.31
White lesions; keratosis

Table 1.14   Causes of oral white lesions

Inflammatory	
Infective	Candidiasis, hairy leukoplakia, syphilitic leukoplakia, Koplik's spots (measles), some papillomas, Reiter's disease, koilocytic dysplasia
Noninfective	Lichen planus, lupus erythematosus
Neoplastic and potentially neoplastic	Leukoplakia, keratoses, carcinoma
Others	Cheek biting, materia alba (debris), burns, grafts, scars, verruciform xanthoma
Congenital	Leukoedema, Fordyce spots, white sponge naevus, focal palmoplantar and oral mucosa hyperkeratosis syndrome, Darier's disease, pachyonychia congenita, dyskeratosis congenita

Most white lesions were formerly known as 'leukoplakia', a term causing misunderstanding and confusion. The World Health Organization defined leukoplakia as a 'white patch or plaque that cannot be characterised clinically or pathologically as any other disease' therefore specifically excluding defined clinicopathological entities such as lichen planus, candidiasis and white sponge naevus, still incorporating white lesions caused by friction or other trauma, and offering no comment on the presence of dysplasia. A subsequent international seminar defined leukoplakia more precisely as 'a whitish patch or plaque that cannot be characterised clinically or pathologically as any other disease and which is not associated with any physical or chemical causative agent except the use of tobacco.'

Diagnosis

The history is important to enable exclusion of a congenital or heredi-tary cause in particular. The clinical appearances may strongly suggest that diagnosis and examination of skin, nails and other sites may be indicated, but investigations are often required if the white lesion does not scrape away from the mucosa with a gauze. Biopsy is then often required.

Management

Treatment is of the underlying cause.

Xerostomia

See Dry Mouth (page 4)

Further reading

Dummett CO. Overview of normal oral pigmentation. *J Indiana Dent Assoc* (1980) **50**: 13–18.

Dummett CO. Pertinent considerations in oral pigmentation. *Br Dent J* (1985) **158**: 9–12.

Porter SR, Scully C. Temporomandibular joint disorders. *Med Int* (1990) **76**: 3170–1.

Scully C. Orofacial manifestations in the rheumatic disorders. *Dent Update* (1989) **16**: 240–6.

Scully C. The Oral Cavity. In: Champion RH, Burton JL, Burns DA, Breathnach SM, eds, *Textbook of Dermatology*, 6th edn. (Blackwells: Oxford, 1998) 3047–123.

Scully C, El-Maaytah M, Greenman J, Porter SR. Breath odor: etiopathogen-esis, assessment and management. *Eur J Oral Sci* (1997) **105**: 287–93.

Scully C, Porter SR, Greenman J. What to do about halitosis. *BMJ* (1994) **308**: 217–18 (editorial).

Orofacial pain with a neurological or vascular background

Pain is the most common oral complaint. Usually it has a local cause, but neurological, vascular, psychogenic and other causes should be excluded (Table 2.1). Pain control is summarised in Table 10.3.

Causalgia

Causalgia is a persistent burning pain, often in the mandible, that follows surgery or trauma. The cause is unclear and there is no good evidence that it is related to a peripheral nerve lesion or to psychogenic causes. If a local analgesic injection temporarily relieves causalgia, then cryoanalgesia may effect more permanent relief, but neurosurgery may ultimately be required.

Cranial arteritis (temporal arteritis; giant-cell arteritis)

Incidence

Rare

Age mainly affected

Elderly

Sex mainly affected

F>M

Table 2.1 Differential diagnosis of orofacial pain

Pain	Dental	Periodontal	Mucosal	Salivary glands	Neuralgic	Vascular	TMJ pain dysfunction	Psychogenic
Location	Mouth, ear, jaws, cheek	Tooth	Mucosa	Area of gland	Nerve distribution	Orbit or upper face	Temple, ear, jaws, teeth	Diffuse, deep, sometimes across midline
Localization	Poor, diffuse, radiating, does not cross midline	Good	Usually good	Usually good	Good	Usually good	Poor, but usually unilateral	Poor
Duration	Seconds to days	Hours to days	Hours to days	Hours to days	Seconds	Minutes to hours	Weeks to years	Weeks to years
Character	Intermittent, sharp, paroxysmal	Steady, boring	Burning or sharp	Drawing, pulling	Lancinating, paroxysmal	Throbbing, deep	Dull, continuous	Dull, boring continuous
Precipitating factors	Hot and cold	Chewing	Sour and spicy foods	Eating	Touch, wind	Alcohol	Yawning, chewing	Stress, fatigue
Associated features	Caries, exposed dentine	Abscess	Erosions or ulcers	Salivary gland swelling	None usually	Lacrimation, injected eye, nasal discharge	Click in TMJ, trismus	None
Aetiology	Caries, trauma, cracked tooth	Acute periodontitis	Varied	Saliva, retention, infection	Idiopathic, multiple sclerosis	Vasomotor	Stress, parafunction	Depression
Management	Restoration endodontics	Peridontics or extraction	According to cause	Drainage, antibiotics	Carbamazepine, nerve block, cryoanalgesia, neurosurgery	Sumatriptan	Antidepressants, other treatments	Antidepressants and psychotherapy

Aetiology

Cranial arteritis appears to be an immunological type of disease affecting middle-sized arteries. Biopsy shows the arterial elastic tissues to be fragmented, with giant cells numerous in the region of the deranged internal elastic lamina.

Clinical features

Cranial arteritis is characterized by:

- Deep and aching, throbbing and persistent unilateral pain;
- Pain often over the temple;
- Pain often made worse when the patient lies flat;
- Pain which may be exacerbated or reduced by pressure on the artery involved;
- Tenderness of the affected superficial temporal and other cranial arteries;
- . Retinal artery involvement which may culminate in blindness;
- Oral pain which may precede ulceration or gangrene (Figure 2.1);
- Systemic features including malaise, weakness, weight loss, anorexia, fever, sweating;
- Raised erythrocyte sedimentation rate.

Diagnosis

The clinical features are fairly diagnostic but it is important to look for a raised erythrocyte sedimentation rate (or plasma viscosity), and a temporal artery biopsy may be indicated.

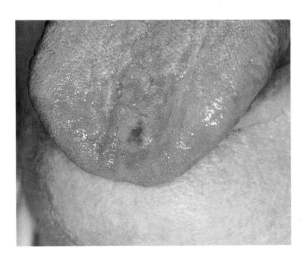

Figure 2.1
Cranial arteritis typically causes pain but may rarely lead to ulceration or gangrene

Management

Patients with cranial arteritis may be threatened with retinal damage and loss of vision, and therefore should be given urgent treatment with systemic corticosteroids (prednisolone 60–80 mg daily).

Frey's syndrome (auriculotemporal syndrome; gustatory sweating)

Definition

This is a paroxysmal burning pain, usually in the temporal area in front of the ear, associated with flushing and sweating on eating.

Incidence

Rare

Age mainly affected

Adults

Sex mainly affected

M=F

Aetiology

Frey's syndrome may follow damage to the neural supply to sweat glands and blood vessels. During nerve regeneration, parasympathetic fibres are misdirected down sympathetic nerve pathways. It is typically seen starting several months after surgery, and is especially common after parotidectomy.

Clinical features

This is a paroxysmal burning pain, usually in the temporal area, associated with flushing and sweating on eating.

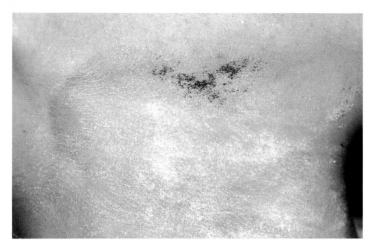

Figure 2.2
Frey's syndrome; positive starch–iodine test

Diagnosis

A starch iodine test confirms sweating in response to a stimulus such as a citrus fruit (Figure 2.2).

Management

20% Aluminium chloride hexahydrate topically

Glossopharyngeal neuralgia

Glossopharyngeal neuralgia affecting the throat and ear is much less common than trigeminal neuralgia (page 49) but the pain is similar, and typically triggered by swallowing or coughing. Occasionally it is secondary to a tumour. Carbamazepine is used, but adequate relief of pain can be difficult.

Herpetic and postherpetic neuralgia

Definition

Neuralgia which persists after herpes zoster (shingles)

Incidence

Uncommon

Age mainly affected

Elderly

Sex mainly affected

M=F

Aetiology

Herpes varicella-zoster virus reactivation

Clinical features

A continuous burning pain that may be so intolerable that suicide can become a risk (Figures 2.3 and 2.4).

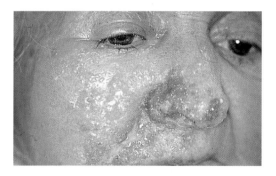

Figure 2.3
Herpes zoster: is preceded, accompanied and often followed by severe orofacial pain

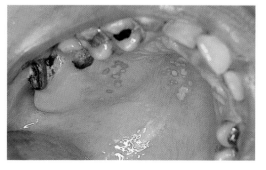

Figure 2.4
Herpes zoster may simulate toothache and this can be a diagnostic problem, when, as here, the patient also has an obvious dental cause for pain

Diagnosis

The history is usually indicative.

Management

Systemic aciclovir, famciclovir or valciclovir used during an attack of zoster can markedly reduce the prevalence of postherpetic neuralgia (Table 10.9). Analgesia is required (Table 10.3) but neuralgia may only respond to tricyclics (Table 10.10), carbamazepine, sodium valproate or topical 0.025% capsaicin.

Migraine

Definition

Migraine is a severe headache associated with nausea and sometimes photophobia (Table 2.2).

Incidence

Uncommon

Age mainly affected

Adult

Sex mainly affected

F>M

Aetiology

Migraine is a headache probably related to arterial dilatation. Attacks may be precipitated by:

- Alcohol;
- Various tyramine-containing foods such as ripe bananas or chocolate;
- Contraceptive pill;
- Stress.

There is no reliable evidence that occlusal problems underlie most migraines.

Table 2.2 Differentiation of important types of facial pain

	Migraine	Migrainous neuralgia	Idiopathic trigeminal neuralgia	Psychogenic
Age of onset	Any	30–50	50	35–60
Gender	F>M	M>F	F>M	F>M
Site	Any	Retro-orbital	Unilateral, mandible or maxilla	Diffuse, deep, sometimes across midline
Associated features	± Photophobia ± Nausea ± Vomiting	± Conjunctival injection ±Lacrimation ± Nasal congestion	—	Life events Back pain etc
Character	Throbbing	Boring	Lancinating	Dull, boring continuous
Duration of episode	Hours (usually day time)	Few hours (usually night time)	Brief (seconds)	Weeks to years
Precipitating factors	± Foods ± Stress	± Alcohol	Trigger areas	Depression
Relieving factors	Sumatriptan; ergot derivatives	Sumatriptan; ergot derivatives; oxygen, indometacin	Carbamazepine	Antidepressants; psychotherapy

Clinical features

Classic migraine has the following features:

- Recurrent headache which is usually severe, unilateral (hemicrania) and lasts for hours or days;
- Preceding warning symptoms (an aura) of visual, sensory, motor or speech disturbances;
- Visual phenomena are often of zig-zag coloured lights (fortification spectra) or transient visual defects;
- Photophobia;
- Nausea or vomiting.

Fortunately, the number, frequency and intensity of attacks usually diminish with increasing age and spontaneous remissions are not uncommon.

Diagnosis

The clinical features are usually indicative.

Management

In acute attacks aspirin or paracetamol may give some relief (Table 10.3). Ergotamine or the $5HT_1$ agonist sumatriptan given early may abort an attack, but should only be prescribed by a physician, since they can produce serious adverse reactions. Naratriptan, rizatriptan and zolmitriptan are claimed to have better absorption than sumatriptan. $5HT_1$ agonists must not be used in patients with cardiac disease. Intranasal lignocaine (lidocaine) may help. Often patients prefer to lie in a quiet, dark room.

Migrainous neuralgia (cluster headache)

Age mainly affected

Young adults

Sex mainly affected

M>F

Aetiology

Migrainous neuralgia is related to vascular changes, and is often precipitated by alcohol.

Clinical features

The pain typically:

- Is localized around the eye;
- Is unilateral;
- Occurs in attacks, which last less than 1 hour, commence and often terminate suddenly;
- Often awakens the patient at night or in the early hours of the morning (2–3 am);
- Is burning and 'boring' in character;
- Is associated on the affected side with the profuse watering of the eye and congestion of the conjunctiva, and nasal discharge and obstruction.

Management

- Alcohol should be avoided;
- Indometacin 75 mg at night may help prevent attacks, as may calcium channel blockers;
- Attacks of migrainous neuralgia are managed, by the physician, with oxygen inhalations, ergotamine or sumatriptan or other $5HT_1$ agonists discussed above.

Neuralgia-inducing cavitational osteonecrosis

Recently described, this rare condition is a hereditary tendency to thrombosis due to:

- Decreased fibrinolysis;
- Disorders of antithrombin; or
- Disorders of protein C.

This may induce small areas of osteonecrosis in bone, including the jaws, resulting in pain. Analgesics, anticoagulation and antimicrobials may be indicated.

Referred pain

Pain may occasionally be referred to the face or jaws from conditions affecting the:

- Neck;
- Lungs;
- Heart.

Anginal pain usually affects the mandible, is initiated by exercise (especially in the cold) and abates quickly on rest.

Trigeminal neuralgia with no obvious neurological cause
(trigeminal neuralgia; idiopathic trigeminal neuralgia; benign paroxysmal trigeminal neuralgia; tic doloureux)

Definition

Orofacial neuralgia in which an organic cause cannot be established

Incidence

Uncommon

Age mainly affected

Elderly

Sex mainly affected

F>M

Aetiology

The cause is unclear, but it may be due to an atherosclerotic blood vessel pressing on the roots of the trigeminal nerve.

Clinical features

Trigeminal neuralgia is the most common neurological cause of orofacial pain. The condition has the following main characteristics.
   Severe pain which typically is:

* Of abrupt onset and termination;
* Electric shock-like, brief, stabbing (lancinating);
* Unilateral;
* Restricted to the trigeminal nerve, usually the mandibular division;
* In some patients triggered by chewing, talking, swallowing, smiling or exposure to temperature change—usually cold air. The

trigger site bears no necessary anatomical relation to the painful area, but is always ipsilateral.

Pain-free intervals between attacks. There may be apparent remissions for months or years, but recurrence is common and over time the pain may spread to a wider area and the intervals between episodes shorten.

No neurological abnormalities. Neurological assessment is needed because similar pain may be secondary to conditions such as:

- Cerebrovascular disease;
- Chronic posttraumatic headache;
- Diseases of the skull;
- Intracranial bleeding;
- Intracranial infections;
- Medical diseases, e.g. neurosyphilis, HIV;
- Meningeal irritation;
- Multiple sclerosis;
- Raised intracranial pressure e.g. cerebral tumour.

Diagnosis

Severe orofacial pain suggestive of trigeminal neuralgia but with physical signs such as facial sensory or motor impairment can result from multiple sclerosis, infections such as HIV infection, or neoplasms. These must therefore be excluded by:

- History;
- Examination;
- Investigations such as CT/MRI.

Management

- Patients with trigeminal neuralgia are best seen at an early stage by a specialist in order to confirm the diagnosis and initiate treatment;
- Medical treatment is used successfully for most patients, typically using anticonvulsants;
- Carbamazepine is still the main anticonvulsant used. It is *not* an analgesic and, if given when an attack starts, will not relieve the pain. It must be given continuously prophylactically for long periods, typically starting with 100 mg three times daily, increasing by 100 mg every 3 days to a maximum of 1000 mg/day, to try to

control the pain while at the same time trying to avoid adverse effects;

- Carbamazepine must be used carefully and under strict medical surveillance since it can have a range of adverse effects, particularly affecting balance, bowels, bone marrow (red and white cells and/or platelets may be depressed) and blood pressure (may increase). Rarely there are severe rashes or dyskinesias;
- Patients should have monthly tests for 3 months, then 6-monthly, of red and white cell and platelet numbers, urea and electrolytes, liver function and blood pressure estimations;
- If carbamazepine fails to control the pain, oxcarbazine, phenytoin, clonazepam, gabapentin or baclofen are occasionally useful;
- If medical treatment fails or the adverse drug effects are too pronounced, surgery may be required.

Local cryosurgery to the trigeminal nerve branches involved (cryoanalgesia) can produce analgesia without permanent anaesthesia, but the benefit can usually be measured only in months rather than years.

For intractable cases, neurosurgery such as destruction of the trigeminal ganglion (radiofrequency ganglionolysis) or decompression of the trigeminal nerve may be required. Unfortunately, pain is exchanged for anaesthesia and risk of damage to the cornea, or occasionally, continuous anaesthesia but with pain (anaesthesia dolorosa).

Further reading

Baillie S, Woodhouse K, Scully C. Medical aspects of ageing: facial and oral pain. In: Barnes IE, Walls A, eds, *Gerodontology* (Wright-Butterworths: Oxford, 1994) 7–16.

Bouquot JE, Roberts AM, Person P et al. Neuralgia-inducing cavitational osteonecrosis (NICO). Osteomyelitis in 224 jawbone samples from patients with facial neuralgia. *Oral Surg Oral Med Oral Pathol* (1992) **73**: 307–19.

Brandt T, Illingworth RD, Peatfield RC. Trigeminal and glossopharyngeal neuralgia. In: Brandt T, Caplan LR, Dichans J et al, eds, *Neurological Disorders: Course and Treatment.* (Academic Press: New York, 1996) 49–58.

Caplan L, Gorelick P. 'Salt and pepper on the face' pain in acute brainstem ischemia. *Ann Neurol* (1983) **13**: 344–5.

Dalessio DJ. Aspirin prophylaxis for migraine. *JAMA* (1990) **264**: 1721.

Diener HC, Peatfield RC. Migraine. In: Brandt T, Caplan LR, Dichans J et al, eds, *Neurological Disorders: Course and Treatment.* (Academic Press: New York, 1996) 1–15.

Dieterich M, Pfaffenrath V. Atypical facial pain. In: Brandt T, Caplan LR, Dichans J et al, eds, *Neurological Disorders: Course and Treatment*. (Academic Press: New York, 1999) 43–7.

Epstein JB, Schubert M, Scully C. Evaluation and treatment of pain in patients with orofacial cancer: a review. *Pain Clinic* (1991) **4**: 3–20.

Greenhall RCD. Headache and facial pain. *Medicine (UK)* (1980) **31**: 1606–10.

Hays LL, Novack AL, Worsham JC. The Frey syndrome: a simple effective treatment. *Otolaryngol Head Neck Surg* (1982) **90**: 419–25.

Henderson WR. Trigeminal neuralgia: the pain and its treatment. *BMJ* (1967) **i**: 7–15.

Illingworth RD. Selective posterior fossa trigeminal nerve section for treatment of trigeminal neuralgia. *Proc R Soc Med* (1974) **67**: 770.

Jannetta PJ. Trigeminal neuralgia and hemifacial spasm: etiology and definitive treatment. *Trans Am Neurol Assoc* (1975) **100**: 89–91.

Kittrelle J, Grouse D, Seybold M. Cluster headaches; local anesthetic abortive agents. *Arch Neurol* (1985) **42**: 496–8.

Klineberg I. *Craniomandibular disorders and orofacial pain*. (Butterworth-Heinemann: Oxford, 1991).

Kost RG, Straus SE. Postherpetic neuralgia: pathogenesis, treatment, and prevention. *N Engl J Med* (1996) **335**: 32–42.

Lazar ML, Greenlee RG, Naarden AL. Facial pain of neurologic origin mimicking oral pathologic conditions; some current concepts and treatment. *J Am Dent Assoc* (1980) **100**: 884–8.

Maizels M, Scott B, Cohen W, Chen W. Intranasal lidocaine for treatment of migraine. *JAMA* (1996) **276**: 319–21.

Olesen J. Classification and diagnostic criteria of headache disorders, cranial neuralgia and facial pain. *Cephalalgia* (1988) **8**: 1–96.

Ratner EJ, Persch P, Kleinman DJ et al. Jawbone cavities and trigeminal and atypical facial neuralgias. *Oral Surg Oral Med Oral Pathol* (1979) **48**: 3–20.

Reutens DC. Burning oral and mid-facial pain in ventral pontine infarction. *Aust NZ J Med* (1990) **20**: 249.

Scully C. The mouth in general practice. 3. Oral and facial pain. *Dermatol Practice* (1982) **1**: 16–18.

Scully C. Oral medicine: pain and neurological disease. In: Bell CJ, ed, *Heinemann Dental Handbook*. (Heinemann: Oxford, 1996) 426–32.

Scully C, Porter SR. Oral Medicine: 4. Orofacial pain. *Postgrad Dent* (1993) **3**: 186–8.

Watkins PJ. Facial sweating after food: a new sign of diabetic autonomic neuropathy. *BMJ* (1973) **i**: 583–587.

3

Orofacial complaints with a significant psychogenic background

The mouth is concerned intimately with the psychological development of the individual and psychogenic complaints are common. Psychogenic orofacial complaints can be seen in:

- Normal persons under stress;
- Persons with a personality trait, such as hypochondriasis;
- Neurotic, often depressed persons;
- Psychotic patients.

Clinical features

Features common to these symptoms are that:

- The patient often appears otherwise quite well;
- Symptoms are chronic, often of a constant type;
- Symptoms may be ill-defined in location or pattern;
- Symptoms do not wake the patient from sleep;
- Adverse life events, such as bereavement or family illness may precede the onset;
- Multiple oral and/or other psychogenic related complaints such as headaches, chronic back pains, irritable bowel syndrome or dysmenorrhoea are common;
- Few of those patients affected seem to try or persist in using treatments offered;
- Many affected persons are middle-aged or older females;
- Objective signs are negative;
- Investigations are negative;
- Multiple consultations are common;

- Cure is uncommon;
- Symptoms may ameliorate on vacations.

It must be stressed that such a diagnosis should be made only where there has been very careful exclusion of organic disease. Many of these patients need to see a specialist since psychiatric assessment may be helpful. Some patients respond to antidepressants such as dothiepin (dosulepin) 75 mg (Table 10.10), but others refuse psychiatric help or medication.

Anorexia nervosa/bulimia

Oral complications may include:

- Tooth erosion from gastric regurgitation;
- Sialosis (Chapter 5);
- Occasionally palatal petechiae or ulceration;
- Manifestations of deficiency states, in the later stages (Chapter 4).

Atypical facial pain

Definition

This term is given to chronic orofacial pain in which no organic cause can be found.

Incidence

Common

Age mainly affected

Middle-aged and elderly

Sex mainly affected

F>M

Aetiology

Over 50% of such patients are depressed or hypochondriacal and though they may blame this on the facial pain, the reverse seems to be true. Many lack insight and will persist in blaming organic diseases for their pain. There appears to be a psychogenic basis in many patients.

Clinical features

Features of atypical facial pain include:

- A dull, continuous ache;
- Location usually in the upper jaw;
- Sleep and appetite are only rarely disturbed;
- Analgesics often appear rarely to have been tried;
- Often, restorative procedures and/or exodontia have been, or are, attempted in vain.

Management

- Organic disease must be carefully excluded;
- The patient should be reassured – although this can be difficult;
- Attempts at relieving pain by restorative treatment, endodontia or exodontia are usually unsuccessful, and the dental surgeon may be blamed for the problem;
- Many patients end up needing to see a specialist, since psychiatric assessment may be helpful;
- Many, however, reject psychiatric advice;
- Some patients respond to antidepressants such as dothiepin (dosulepin), amitriptyline or fluoxetine (Table 15.10), but others refuse drugs.

Atypical odontalgia

Pain and hypersensitive teeth indistinguishable from pulpitis or periodontitis but occurring in the absence of detectable pathology, and aggravated by dental intervention, characterize this disorder. It is probably a variant of atypical facial pain, and should be treated similarly.

Bad taste

See Chapter 1

Burning mouth syndrome
(glossopyrosis; glossodynia; oral dysaesthesia)

Definition

This is a chronic complaint that the mouth has a burning sensation.

Incidence

Common

Age mainly affected

Middle-aged or elderly

Sex mainly affected

F>M

Aetiology

In about 50% of cases, defined local factors which may be at play (Table 3.1) include:
- Tongue-thrusting (Figure 3.1);
- Restricted tongue space from poor denture construction.

In about 30%, there are underlying systemic problems such as:

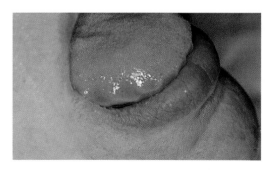

Figure 3.1
Tongue thrusting causing a crenated lateral margin but no obvious organic disease

Table 3.1   Causes of burning mouth

Xerostomia	
Mucosal disorders	Erythema migrans (geographic tongue), lichen planus, infections (candidiasis)
Systemic disease	Deficiencies of vitamins B, folic acid or iron, diabetes mellitus, tertiary syphilis
Psychogenic	Cancerophobia, depression, anxiety states, hypochondriasis
Drugs	Angiotensin converting enzyme inhibitors, gold, erythromycin, coumarins, lithium, chloroquine, protease inhibitors
Foods and drinks	Peanuts, sorbic acid, nicotinic acid, propylglycol

- Haematological deficiency state;
- Diabetes;
- Mucosal disease.

In about 20%, a psychogenic cause is present such as:

- Anxiety;
- Depression;
- Cancerophobia.

Clinical features

Burning mouth syndrome not related to organic oral disease:

- Most frequently affects the tongue, sometimes the palate or less commonly the lips or lower alveolus;
- is usually bilateral;
- is associated with no clinical signs of disease (Figure 3.2);
- is often relieved by eating and drinking, in contrast to pain caused by organic lesions which is typically made worse by food.

Three types have been described (Table 3.2); type 2 is most common, type 3 least common.

Table 3.2   Types of burning mouth syndrome

Type	Symptom pattern	Other features
1	No burning mouth syndrome on waking, but increases during the day	Unremitting
2	Burning mouth syndrome on waking and through the day	Unremitting, difficult to control
3	No regular pattern	May remit

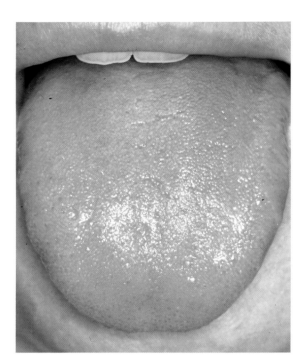

Figure 3.2
Burning mouth syndrome with no clinical evidence of disease

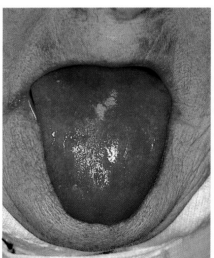

Figure 3.3
Glossitis: may cause discomfort like burning mouth syndrome

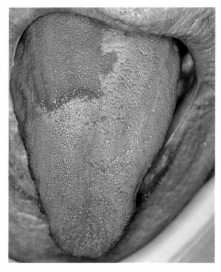

Figure 3.4
Erythema migrans: may cause discomfort like burning mouth syndrome

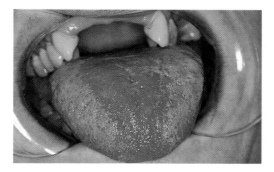

Figure 3.5
Candidiasis: may cause discomfort like burning mouth syndrome

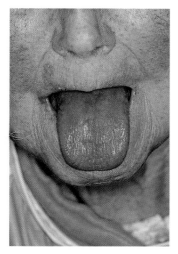

Figure 3.6
Xerostomia: may cause discomfort like burning mouth syndrome, with or without evidence of candidiasis

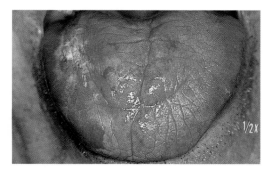

Figure 3.7
Lichen planus: may cause discomfort like burning mouth syndrome

Diagnosis

It is important to do the following:

- Clinically exclude organic causes of discomfort such as glossitis, erythema migrans (geographic tongue), candidiasis, xerostomia or lichen planus (Figure 3.3–3.7);
- Complete a Hospital Anxiety and Depression scale (HAD scale); a score of below 8 is normal but over 10 suggests the need for a psychiatric opinion;
- Undertake laboratory tests to exclude anaemia, a vitamin or iron deficiency (blood tests), diabetes (blood and urine analyses) or candidiasis (oral rinse).

Management

- Any organic cause should be treated;
- Very occasionally a new denture is indicated;
- Reassure the patient;
- It may be helpful empirically to try a 4-week course of vitamin B1 300 mg and vitamin B6 50 mg, three times daily, as a placebo.

Where there is no response, psychiatric care and/or psychoactive drugs may be indicated. If anxiety predominates, dothiepin (dosulepin) 75–150 mg at night may be helpful, and where depression predominates fluoxetine 20 mg at night may be better (Table 10.10). Alpha-lipoic acid or clozapine may be of some value.

Dry mouth

See Chapter 1 (page 4)

Eagle Syndrome

Atypical facial pain may present with throat discomfort which when associated with a prominent styloid process has been termed Eagle Syndrome.

Munchausen Syndrome

This is a rare psychiatric disorder in which patients lie in order to bring about unnecessary investigations and operative treatments.

Syndrome of oral complaints

Multiple pains and other complaints such as dry mouth or bad taste may occur simultaneously or sequentially in this condition, and patients may bring diaries of their symptoms to emphasize their problem. This has been termed the 'maladie du petite papier', and though there is not always a psychogenic basis, such notes characterize patients with non-organic complaints. Relief is rarely admitted. Probably a variant of atypical facial pain, it should be treated similarly.

Temporomandibular pain-dysfunction syndrome
(TMPD; myofascial pain-dysfunction; facial arthromyalgia)

Definition

TMPD is the term given to symptoms such as discomfort, limited mouth opening and/or click related to the temporomandibular joint (TMJ) in persons in whom no organic cause reliably can be identified.

Incidence

Common

Age mainly affected

Adolescents and young adults

Sex mainly affected

F>M

Aetiology

The cause is not clear and has been variously attributed to trauma, occlusal abnormalities, habits or stress. In any event, the underlying cause of discomfort appears to be muscle tension leading to an ischaemic type of pain.

Clinical features

TMPD refers to any or all of the following triad:

- Pain: typically mild and dull and over one side of the face or joint but can radiate elsewhere;
- Limitation of jaw opening: in some there may even be locking;
- Clicking or crepitus from the TMJ: on opening or closing the mouth.

There appear to be no long-term sequelae such as arthritis.

Diagnosis

In all cases, organic disease must first be carefully excluded; similar manifestations have been seen in malignant disease, for example.

Management

There is no defined treatment, and therapies have included the following: rest; use of occlusal splints; occlusal re-equilibration; anxiolytics; antidepressants; analgesics; exercises; short-wave diathermy; acupuncture; lasers; and surgery.

In the absence of any evidence that intervention is indicated or significantly effective, it seems prudent to:

- Counsel rest;
- Possibly use an occlusal splint, at night in the first instance.

Certainly, the majority of patients respond well to this regimen, though some need antidepressant medication (Table 10.10).

Tension headaches

Definition

Tension headaches are stress-related pains in the forehead, temple and/or neck.

Incidence

Common

Age mainly affected

Young adults

Sex mainly affected

M>F

Aetiology

Tension headaches are caused by anxiety or stress-induced muscle tension, presumably because the accumulation of metabolites in the tense muscles produces pain.

Clinical features

The pain affects the upper face (frontal or temporal muscles) or neck (occipital muscles), and not the mouth. Typically it is felt as a constant ache or band-like pressure, often worse by the evening. However, tension headaches do not waken the patient.

Diagnosis

The history and clinical features are indicative. The affected muscles may be tender to palpation; pain may be relieved by massage of these muscles. No diagnostic tests are available.

Management

Reassurance may be effective, but the pain may be helped by relaxation, or anxiolytics such as a little alcohol or benzodiazepines. A change to a more relaxed lifestyle may be indicated.

Further reading

Abrams RA, Ruff JC. Oral signs and symptoms in the diagnosis of bulimia. *J Am Dent Assoc* (1986) **113**: 761–64.

Aghabeigi B, Feinmann C, Harris M. (1992) Prevalence of post-traumatic stress disorder in patients with chronic orofacial pain: pathophysiology and clinical presentation idiopathic facial pain. *Br J Oral Maxillofac Surg* (1992) **30**: 360–64.

Baillie S, Woodhouse K, Scully C. Medical aspects of ageing: facial and oral pain. In: Barnes IE, Walls A, eds, *Gerodontology.* (Oxford: Wright-Butterworths, 1994) 7–16.

Bonica JJ. General considerations of chronic pain. In: Bonica JJ, ed, *The Management of Pain.* (Lea & Febiger: Philadelphia, 1990) 180–3.

Clark DC. Oral complications of anorexia nervosa and/or bulimia. *J Oral Med* (1985) **40**: 134–8.

Epstein JB, Schubert M, Scully C. Evaluation and treatment of pain in patients with orofacial cancer: a review. *Pain Clinic* (1991) **4**: 3–20.

Feinmann C, Harris M. Psychogenic facial pain. The clinical presentation. *Br Dent J* (1984) **156**: 165–9.

Feinmann C, Harris M. Psychogenic facial pain: management and prognosis. *Br Dent J* (1984) **156**: 205–208.

Feinmann C, Harris M, Cawley R. Psychogenic facial pain: presentation and management. *BMJ* (1984) **228**: 436–8.

Fields HL, ed, *Pain Syndromes in Neurology.* (Butterworths: London, 1990).

Friedlander AH, West LJ Dental management of the patient with major depression. *Oral Surg* (1991) **71**: 573–8.

Goodwin FK, Jamieson KR. *Manic-depressive Illness.* (Oxford University Press: Oxford, 1990).

Gram LF. *N Engl J Med* (1994) **331**: 1354–61.

Gross KB, Brough KM, Randolph PM. Eating disorders: anorexia and bulimia nervosa. *ASOC J Dent Child* (1986) **53**: 378–81.

Harris M, Davies G. Psychiatric disorders. In: Jones JH, Mason DK, eds, *Oral Manifestations of Systemic Disease*, 2nd edn. (Baillière Tindall: London, 1990).

Heloe B, Heiberg AN. A follow-up study of a group of female patients with myofascial-pain-dysfunction syndrome. *Acta Odontol Scand* (1980) **38**: 129–34.

Hugoson A, Thorstensson B. Vitamin B status and response to replacement therapy in patients with burning mouth syndrome. *Acta Odontol Scand* (1991) **49**: 367–75.

Johnson GFS, Wilson P. The management of depression: a review of pharmacological and non-pharmacological treatments. *Med J Aust* (1989) **151**: 397–406.

Kane JM, McGlashan TH. Treatment of schizophrenia. *Lancet* (1995) **346**: 820–5.

Kiloh LG. The diagnosis and management of depressive illness. *Medicine (UK)* (1980) **35**: 1773–6.

Klineberg I. *Craniomandibular disorders and orofacial pain.* (Butterworth-Heinemann: Oxford, 1991).

von Knorring L. The pathogenesis of chronic pain syndromes. *Nord Psykiatr Tidsskr* (1989) **43** (Supplement 20): 35–43.

Lamey PJ, Hammond A, Allam BF, McIntosh WB. Vitamin status of patients with burning mouth syndrome. *Br Dent J* (1986) **160**: 81–4.

Lefer L. A psychoanalytic view of a dental phenomenon psychosomatics of the temporomandibular joint pain-dysfunction syndrome. *Contemp Psychiatr* (1966) **2**: 135–50.

Lupton DE. Psychological aspects of temporomandibular joint dysfunction. *J Am Dent Assoc* (1969) **79**: 131–6.

Marbach JJ, Lennon MC, Dohrenwend BP. Candidate risk factors for temporomandibular pain and dysfunction syndrome: psychosocial, health behaviour, physical illness and injury. *Pain* (1988) **34**: 139–51.

Melzack R, Wall PD. *The Challenge of Pain.* (Pelican: London, 1988).

Michels R, Marzuk PM. Progress in Psychiatry (1) and (2). *N Engl J Med* (1993) **329**: 552–60 and 628–38.

Moulton RE. Emotional factors in non-organic temporomandibular joint pain. *Dent Clin North Am* (1966) **Nov**: 609–20.

Pullinger AG, Seligman DA, Gombein JA. A multiple logistic regression analysis of the risk and relative odds of temporomandibular disorders as a function of common occlusal features. *J Dent Res* (1993) **72**: 968–79.

Raphael KG, Dohrenwend BP, Marbach JJ. Illness and injury among children of temporomandibular pain and dysfunction syndrome (TMPDS) patients. *Pain* (1990) **40**: 61–4.

Schiffman E, Fricton JR. Epidemiology of TMJ and craniofacial pain. In: Fricton JR, Kroening RJ, Hathaway KM, eds, *TMJ and Craniofacial Pain. Diagnosis and Management.* (EuroAmerica: St Louis, 1989)

Scully C. La maladie du petit papier. *Br Dent J* (1993) **175**: 289–92.

Scully C, Porter SR. Oral medicine: 4. Orofacial pain. *Postgrad Dent* (1993) **3**: 186–8.

Scully C, Eveson JW, Porter SR. Munchausen's syndrome: oral presentations. *Br Dent J* (1995) **178**, 65–7.

Sessle BJ. The neurology of facial and dental pain: present knowledge, future directions. *J Dent Res* (1987) **66**: 962–81.

Southwell J, Deary IJ, Geissler P. Personality and anxiety in temporo-mandibular joint syndrome patients. *J Oral Rehabil* (1990) **17**: 239–43.

Speculand B, Hughes AO, Gross AN. Role of stressful life experiences in the onset of TMJ pain dysfunction. *Community Dent Oral Epidemiol* (1984) **12**: 197–202.

Stiefel DJ, Truelove EL, Menard TW et al. A comparison of the oral health of persons with and without chronic mental illness in community settings. *Spec Care Dentist* (1990) **10**: 6–12.

Strauss JS, Carpenter WT. *Schizophrenia.* (Plenum Press: New York, 1981).

Toller PA. Temporomandibular joint arthropathy. *Proc R Soc Med* (1974) **67**: 153–9.

Van der Waal I. *The Burning Mouth Syndrome.* (Munksgaard: Copenhagen, 1990).

Walsh BT, Croft CB, Katz JL. Anorexia nervosa and salivary gland enlargement. *Int J Psychiatry Med* (1981) **11**: 255–61.

Woodforde JM, Merskey H. Personality traits of patients with chronic pain. *J Psychosom Res* (1972) **16**: 167–72.

4

Mucosal disorders

The mucosa is divided into masticatory, lining and specialized types. Masticatory mucosa (hard palate, gingiva), is adapted to the forces of pressure and friction and keratinized with numerous tall rete ridges and connective tissue papillae and little submucosa. Lining mucosa (buccal, labial and alveolar mucosa, floor of mouth, ventral surface of tongue, soft palate, lips) is nonkeratinized and relatively mobile, with broad rete ridges and connective tissue papillae and abundant elastic fibres in the lamina propria.

Specialized mucosa on the dorsum of the tongue, adapted for taste and mastication, is keratinized, with numerous rete ridges and connective tissue papillae, abundant elastic and collagen fibres in the lamina propria and no submucosa. The tongue bears numerous papillae on the dorsum mainly; they include circumvallate (at the junction of anterior two-thirds and posterior tongue), foliate (at the posterolateral margin), fungiform and filiform papillae (scattered over the anterior dorsum). A frenulum connects the anterior ventrum to the floor of mouth, and plicae fimbriata run down the ventrum bilaterally (Table 4.1).

Terms used in the description of oral pathology are shown in Tables 4.2 and 4.3.

Acanthosis nigricans

This is a rare condition characterized by pigmented velvety plaques on the:

- Neck;
- Popliteal region;
- Antecubital fossae;
- Periumbilically.

Table 4.1   Epithelia in different oral locations

Epithelium	Mucosal site
Nonkeratinized	Buccal, labial and vestibules, tongue lateral and ventral, floor of mouth, soft palate
Orthokeratinized	Gingivae, tongue dorsal, hard palate, alveolar
Parakeratinized	Gingivae, tongue dorsal, alveolar

Table 4.2   Descriptive clinical terms used for mucosal and other lesions

Term	Meaning
Angioedema	Diffuse swelling appearing acutely
Asboe–Hansen sign	Blister spreads under pressure
Atrophy	Thinning
Blister	Fluid filled lesions
Bulla	Blister >5 mm diameter
Erosion	Partial loss of epithelium
Erythema	Redness
Fissure	Linear ulcer
Koebner phenomenon	Trauma results in new lesions
Macule	Flat lesion <1 cm diameter
Nikolsky sign	Minor trauma induces a blister
Nodule	Raised lesion >1 cm diameter
Papule	Raised lesion <1 cm diameter
Plaque	Large flattish lesion (>1 cm diameter)
Pustule	Blister containing pus
Rhagade	Deep fissure
Ulcer	Loss of epithelium extending to lamina propria
Vesicle	Blister <5 mm diameter

Table 4.3   Histopathological terms in common usage

Term	Meaning
Acantholysis	Cell separation in the stratum spinosum
Acanthosis	Thickening of the stratum spinosum (leads to broadened longer rete pegs)
Pseudoepitheliomatous hyperplasia	Extremely elongated rete pegs giving the false appearance of carcinoma: the epithelium is not dysplastic
Hyperkeratosis	Excessive thickening of the cornified layer
Orthokeratin	Nonnucleated keratin
Parakeratin	Nucleated cornified layer, with pyknotic nuclei

It may be congenital, or acquired and then usually associated with:

- Malignancy (mainly glandular adenocarcinomas such as gastric, but also tumours in the uterus, liver, colon, rectum, or ovaries);
- Diabetes mellitus;
- Drug use.

Oral lesions are not usually seen in hereditary forms but are seen in 50% of those with acquired acanthosis nigricans, manifesting with nonpigmented:

- Macroglossia;
- Cobblestoned buccal mucosa;
- Gingival swelling;
- Commissural plaque-like lesions.

Acrodermatitis enteropathica

Acrodermatitis enteropathica is a rare autosomal dominant condition of impaired zinc absorption. It manifests from infancy with:

- Vesiculobullous skin lesions;
- Alopecia;
- Diarrhoea;
- Oral lesions, including angular stomatitis, ulcers and erythematous lesions.

Addison's disease

Definition

Addison's disease is adrenocortical hypofunction. It results in hypotension and a feedback pituitary overproduction of adrenocorticotrophic hormone (ACTH) that produces hyperpigmentation of skin and mucosae.

Incidence

Rare

Age mainly affected

Young and middle-aged

Sex mainly affected

F>M

Aetiology

Addison's disease is due to adrenocortical damage and hypofunction, usually autoimmune, but rare causes include tuberculosis, carcinomatosis and histoplasmosis (sometimes in AIDS). Nelson's syndrome is similar but iatrogenic and results from adrenalectomy in the management of breast cancer.

Clinical features

Hyperpigmentation is generalized and brown, most obvious in areas normally pigmented such as:

- Areolae of nipples;
- Genitalia;
- Skin flexures;
- Sites of trauma.

The oral mucosa may show patchy or diffuse brown hyperpigmentation (Figure 4.1). Other features of Addison's disease include:

- Weakness;
- Anorexia;
- Weight loss;
- Low blood pressure;
- Collapse under stress.

Diagnosis

It may be necessary to differentiate racial from drug-induced and other causes of hyperpigmentation. It is important to establish

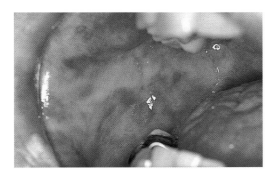

Figure 4.1
Addison's disease

whether there is adrenal hypofunction, and the cause. Adrenal hypofunction is established if:

- Blood pressure is reduced;
- Plasma cortisol levels are reduced;
- Response to ACTH stimulation (Synacthen test using adrenocorticotropic hormone [ACTH]) is reduced.

Management

Addison's disease is treated by replacement therapy with fludrocortisone and corticosteroids.

Amalgam and other tattoos

Definition

Amalgam or other foreign materials incorporated into a wound may cause a tattoo.

Incidence

Common

Age mainly affected

After adolescence

Sex mainly affected

M=F

Aetiology

Amalgam or dust can become incorporated in healing wounds after tooth extraction or apicectomy or beneath mucosa. Similar lesions can result if pencil lead (graphite) or other similar foreign bodies become embedded in the oral tissues. Occasionally adolescents may deliberately have tattoos made in their mouth.

Clinical features

Tattoos usually:

- Are blue-black spots or macules (Figure 4.2);

- Do not grow in size;
- Are usually seen close to the teeth if caused by amalgam (Figure 4.3);
- Are often in the buccal mandibular gingiva (Figure 4.4), the floor of the mouth, or the scar of an apicectomy where there has been a retrograde root-filling if caused by amalgam (Figure 4.5);
- May be in the palate if caused by graphite (Figure 4.6);
- May occasionally show opacities on radiography.

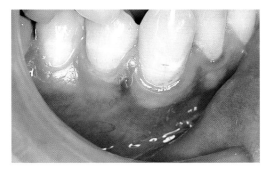

Figure 4.2
Amalgam tattoo in a typical site

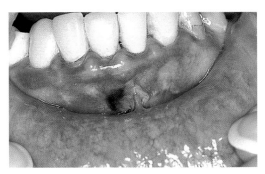

Figure 4.3
Amalgam tattoo after apicectomy

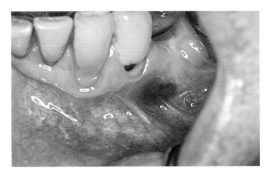

Figure 4.4
Amalgam tattoo

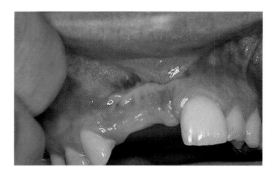

Figure 4.5
Amalgam tattoo

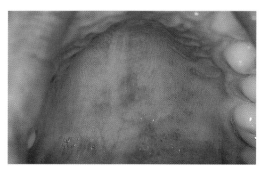

Figure 4.6
Graphite tattoo from a childhood accident involving a pencil penetrating the palatal mucosa

Diagnosis

- The diagnosis is usually obvious from the location, history and clinical appearance;
- Radiography may or may not help to confirm the diagnosis;
- Biopsy may be indicated in cases where the clinical diagnosis is equivocal, in order to exclude a naevus or melanoma, but otherwise these lesions are innocuous.

Management

- These lesions can be left alone if the diagnosis is certain;
- Those rare tattoos which need removal for cosmetic reasons can be excised or removed with a Q-switched ruby laser.

Amyloid

See Chapter 9

Aphthae (recurrent aphthous stomatitis, RAS; Tables 4.4 and 4.5)

Definition

RAS are recurrent mouth ulcers which typically start in childhood and have a natural history to improve with age (Figure 4.7).

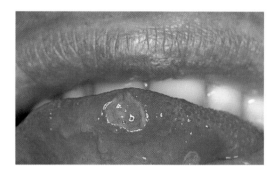

Figure 4.7
Recurrent aphthous stomatitis

Incidence

RAS affect up to 25% of the population.

Table 4.4   Characteristics of the different types of recurrent aphthous stomatitis

	Minor	Major	Herpetiform
Sex ratio	M=F	M=F	F>M
Age of onset (years)	10–19	10–19	20–29
Number	1–5	1–10	10–100
Diameter (mm)	<10	>10	1–2
Duration (days)	4–14	>30	>30
Rate of recurrence (months)	1–4	<Monthly	<Monthly
Locations			
Lips	+	+	+
Cheeks	+	+	+
Tongue	–	+	+
Palate	–	+	+
Scarring after ulceration	–	+	+/–

Age mainly affected

Children and young adults

Sex mainly affected

M=F

Aetiology

There may be:

- A family history;
- Associations with HLA-antigens B51 and Cw7;
- Changes in cell-mediated immune responses and cross-reactivity with *Streptococcus sanguis* or heat shock protein.

There appears to be a genetically determined immunological reactivity to unidentified antigens, possibly microbial. Research has shown equivocal associations with various viruses (cytomegalovirus, varicella-zoster virus, herpes simplex virus), and other microorganisms (streptococci, *Helicobacter pylori*). Immunological changes are detectable, but there is no reliable evidence of autoimmune disease (Figures 4.8–4.12).

Most patients with RAS are well, but some prove to have associations with:

- Stress;
- Trauma;
- Deficiency of a haematinic such as iron, folate or vitamin B12 (about 10–20%), or B1;
- Coeliac disease or Crohn's disease;
- Menstruation;
- Food allergy: some react to nuts, chocolate, potato crisps, etc.

Aphthae are less common in smokers than in nonsmokers, and sometimes they appear when smokers give up the habit.

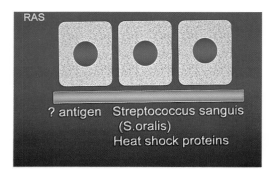

Figure 4.8
Recurrent aphthous stomatitis: an immunological reaction to various antigens eventually damages keratinocytes and epithelial basement membrane

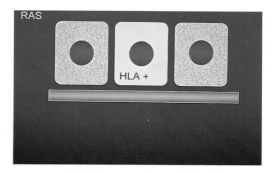

Figure 4.9
Recurrent aphthous stomatitis: keratinocytes express HLA antigens at an early stage

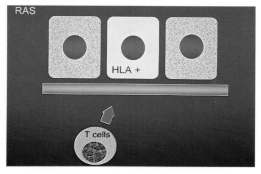

Figure 4.10
Recurrent aphthous stomatitis: T lymphocytes move into early lesion

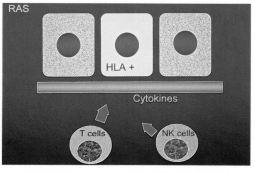

Figure 4.11
Recurrent aphthous stomatitis: cytokines from T lymphocytes attract natural killer cells

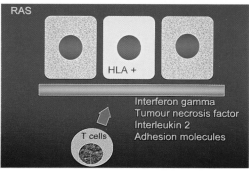

Figure 4.12
Recurrent aphthous stomatitis: multiple cytokines appear involved in pathogenesis of damage to keratinocytes

A small minority of patients prove to have systemic disease such as:

- Behçet's syndrome;
- Immunodeficiencies, including HIV disease, IgG_2 deficiency and cyclic neutropenia;
- A syndrome with periodic fever and pharyngitis (page 33), but with no neutropenia;
- Cytophagic histiocytic panniculitis;
- Sweet's syndrome.

Clinical features

Recurrent aphthae typically:

- Start in childhood or adolescence;
- Are multiple (Figure 4.13);
- Are ovoid or round (Figure 4.14);
- Recur;
- Have a yellowish depressed floor (Figure 4.15);
- Have a pronounced red inflammatory halo (Figure 4.16).

Aphthae may present different clinical appearances and behaviours (Table 4.4).

Minor aphthae (Mikulicz's aphthae; MiRAS) are recurrent, often ovoid ulcers with an inflammatory halo, and:

- are small, 2–4 mm in diameter;
- Last 7–10 days;
- Tend not to be seen on gingiva, palate or dorsum of tongue (Figures 4.17 and 4.18);
- Heal with no obvious scarring (Figure 4.19).

Most patients develop not more than six minor ulcers at any single episode.

Major aphthae (Sutton's ulcers; MaRAS) are recurrent, often ovoid ulcers with an inflammatory halo, but are less common, much larger (Figure 4.20) and more persistent than minor aphthae, and can affect the soft palate (Figures 4.21 and 4.22) and dorsum of tongue as well as other sites. Sometimes termed periadenitis mucosa necrotica recurrens (PMNR), major aphthae:

- Can be well over 1 cm in diameter;
- Are most common on the soft palate, fauces and lips;
- Can take several months to heal (Figure 4.23);
- May leave obvious scars on healing (Figures 4.24 and 4.25).

At any one episode there are usually fewer than six ulcers present.

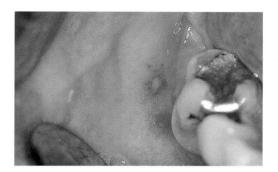

Figure 4.13
*Recurrent aphthous
stomatitis, these are
often small multiple
ulcers*

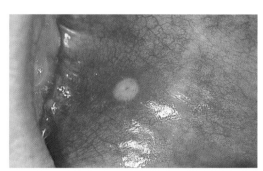

Figure 4.14
*Recurrent aphthous
stomatitis: ulcers are
round or ovoid with an
inflammatory halo*

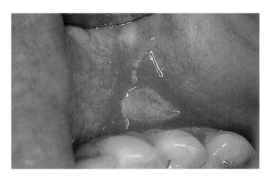

Figure 4.15
*Recurrent aphthous
stomatitis: ulcers have a
yellowish floor*

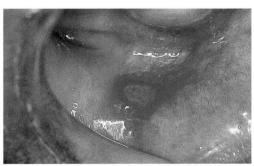

Figure 4.16
*Recurrent aphthous
stomatitis: ulcers have a
surrounding
inflammatory halo*

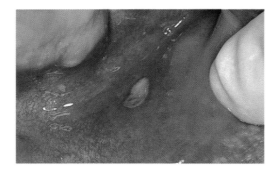

Figure 4.17
*Recurrent aphthous
stomatitis: minor aphthae
in a typical site*

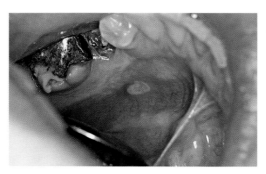

Figure 4.18
*Recurrent aphthous
stomatitis: minor aphthae
affect mobile non-
keratinised mucosa*

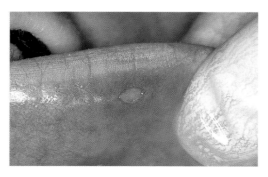

Figure 4.19
*Recurrent aphthous
stomatitis: healing minor
aphthous ulcer*

Herpetiform ulcers (HU) are so termed because the patients have a myriad of small ulcers that clinically resemble those of herpetic stomatitis (Figure 4.26). It is, however, a distinct entity, lacking the associated fever, gingivitis and lymph node involvement of primary herpetic stomatitis. HU are more common in females and:

- Start as multiple pinpoint aphthae;
- Enlarge and fuse to produce irregular ulcers (Figure 4.27);
- Can be seen on any mucosa, but especially on the ventrum of the tongue (Figure 4.28).

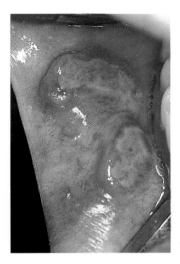

Figure 4.20
Recurrent aphthous stomatitis: major aphthae are large and persistent

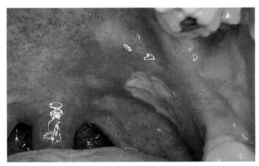

Figure 4.21
Recurrent aphthous stomatitis: major aphthae may affect the palate and tongue

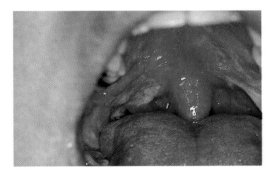

Figure 4.22
Recurrent aphthous stomatitis: major aphthae are large, persistent and can affect any site

Diagnosis

Aphthae are diagnosed from the history and clinical features. There is no diagnostic test of value but blood tests may be useful for excluding

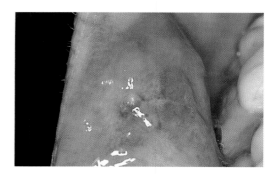

Figure 4.23
Recurrent aphthous stomatitis: persistent major aphthae

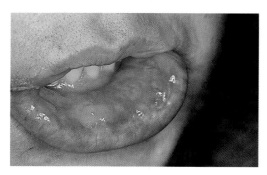

Figure 4.24
Recurrent aphthous stomatitis: scarring after major aphthae

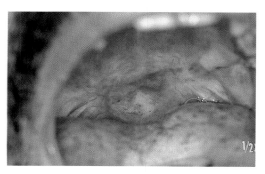

Figure 4.25
Recurrent aphthous stomatitis: severe scarring from major aphthae in this patient with Behçet's syndrome

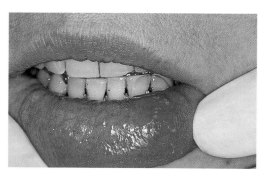

Figure 4.26
Recurrent aphthous stomatitis: herpetiform ulcers are multiple and small initially

possible deficiencies or other conditions, and then a specialist opinion may be of help. Features that might suggest a systemic background, and indicate the need for specialist referral, include:

Any suggestion of systemic disease from extraoral features such as:
- Genital lesions;
- Skin lesions;
- Ocular lesions;
- Gastrointestinal complaints (e.g. pain, altered bowel habits, blood in faeces);
- Loss of weight;
- Weakness;
- Chronic cough;
- Fever;
- Lymphadenopathy;
- Hepatomegaly;
- Splenomegaly;

An atypical history such as:
- Onset of ulcers in later adult life;
- Exacerbation of ulceration;

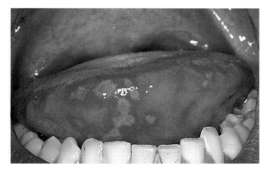

Figure 4.27
Recurrent aphthous stomatitis: herpetiform ulcers fuse to produce ragged lesions

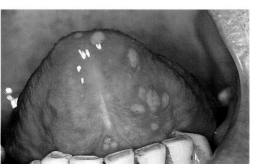

Figure 4.28
Recurrent aphthous stomatitis: herpetiform ulcers often affect the ventrum of the tongue

- Severe aphthae;
- Aphthae unresponsive to topical hydrocortisone or triamcinolone.

Presence of other oral lesions, especially:
- Candidiasis (including angular stomatitis);
- Glossitis;
- Purpura or gingival bleeding;
- Gingival swelling;
- Necrotizing gingivitis;
- Herpetic lesions;
- Hairy leukoplakia;
- Kaposi's sarcoma.

Management

The aims of treatment of RAS are to reduce pain, reduce ulcer duration and increase disease-free intervals. There is no absolute cure.

Any underlying predisposing factors should be treated and, where possible, allergens and irritant foods such as potato crisps should be avoided. Treat aphthae with:

- Benzydamine rinse or spray to ease the discomfort (Table 10.2);
- Chlorhexidine 0.2% aqueous mouthwash (Table 10.1);
- Topical corticosteroids such as hydrocortisone hemisuccinate 2.5 mg pellets or 0.1% triamcinolone acetonide in Orabase used four times daily or, rarely, more potent topical corticosteroids (e.g. betamethasone, beclomethasone or fluticasone (Table 10.5));
- In adults, tetracycline rinses using 250 mg capsules in water four times daily for up to 4 weeks.

Other agents such as thalidomide or immunosuppressive agents are effective and may be needed, but these should be given by a physician, since there may be serious adverse effects (Table 10.7). A range of other agents have appeared effective in small trials but hard evidence of their efficacy is lacking (Table 4.5).

Aspergillosis

Definition

A deep mycosis (fungal infection) caused by *Aspergillus* species, the most common fungi in the environment, being prolific saprophytes in soil and decaying vegetation.

Table 4.5   Some therapies for RAS

Topical corticosteroids	Hydrocortisone hemisuccinate, triamcinolone acetonide, fluocinonide, fluticasone, betamethasone valerate, betamethasone-17-benzoate, flumetasone pivolate, beclomethasone dipropionate
Antimicrobials	Topical tetracyclines, deoxymycine, chlorhexidine gluconate
Immunomodulators	Levamisole, transfer factor, colchicine, gammaglobulins, azathioprine, dapsone, cyclosporin, tacrolimus thalidomide, pentoxifylline, systemic corticosteroids
Others of equivocal efficacy	Benzydamine hydrochloride, carbenoxolone disodium, sucralfate, amlexanox, azelastine, systemic zinc sulphate, monoamine oxidase inhibitors, sodium cromoglycate, etretinate, low-energy laser

Incidence

Uncommon. Aspergillosis is found worldwide, is increasing especially in immunocompromised persons, and is the most prevalent mycosis second only to candidiasis.

Age mainly affected

Adults

Sex mainly affected

M=F

Aetiology

Aspergillus fumigatus is the most common pathogen, but *A. flavus* the most virulent. *A. glaucus, A. nidulans, A. terres, A. repens, A parasiticus* and *A. niger* are also encountered.

Clinical features

Inhalation of the conidiospores must be extremely common, but clinical disease is rare, unless there is massive inhalation or the host is immunocompromised. Aspergillus spores can germinate in mucus and may therefore colonize the respiratory tract to produce the following:

- **Allergic bronchopulmonary aspergillosis**, the most common respiratory disease, typically caused by *A. fumigatus*;
- **Invasive aspergillosis**, which affects the lungs mainly but may spread to brain, bone or endocardium;
- **Aspergillomas**, which are fungus balls that grow in pre-existing cavities such as tuberculous lung cavities or the paranasal sinuses.

Orofacial lesions include the following:

- Antral aspergilloma presenting in a chronically obstructed sinus in an otherwise healthy host;
- Invasive aspergillosis of the antrum seen mainly in immunocompromised hosts. Destruction of the antral wall, with antral pain, swelling or sequelae from orbital invasion (impaired ocular motility, exophthalmos, or impaired vision), or intracranial extension (headaches, meningism) are typical features;
- Indolent chronic sinusitis; defects in cell-mediated immune responses to aspergillus often underlie sinus aspergillosis, although occasional cases result from metastasis from pulmonary aspergillosis or arise iatrogenically following extractions, endodontics or implants involving the antrum;
- Allergic sinusitis;
- Oral lesions which present as yellow or black, necrotic ulcers, typically in the palate or occasionally the posterior tongue.

Diagnosis

- MR and CT imaging are more sensitive than conventional radiography in detecting bone erosion in invasive aspergillosis;
- Diagnosis is confirmed by smear and lesional microscopy. Culture of tissue or fluids may be positive but not invariably. Isolation of aspergillus is not *proof* of disease since the organisms are ubiquitous;
- Estimations of serum precipitins and IgE specific antibody may support the diagnosis.

Management

Non-invasive antral aspergillosis: antral debridement and restoration of drainage.
Invasive aspergillosis: surgical debridement, intravenous amphotericin and hyperbaric oxygen.
Oral aspergillosis: systemic amphotericin, fluconazole or itraconazole (Table 10.8).

Behçet's syndrome (Behçet's disease: Adamantiades syndrome)

Definition

Aphthae associated with systemic disease manifesting usually with genital ulcers and uveitis

Incidence

This is a rare condition, most common in Japan, China, Korea and the Middle East (along the ancient silk route from Europe to the Far East).

Age mainly affected

Young adults

Sex mainly affected

M>F

Aetiology

Behçet's syndrome appears to have:

- An immunogenetic basis, with a specific but weak association with HLA-B5 (B5101);
- Immunological changes like those in aphthae;
- Immune complexes, possibly with herpes simplex virus;
- Cytokine involvement (interleukins, tumour necrosis factor);
- An association with heat shock proteins (hsp);
- Hyperactive polymorphonuclear leukocytes (Figures 4.29–4.31).

Clinical features

Behçet's syndrome is a multisystem disease affecting the mouth in most cases (Figure 4.32) with aphthous-like ulcers affecting the palate especially and often being persistent. Many other sites are commonly affected.

   Genitals: Ulcers resembling oral aphthae affect the scrotum and labia majora mainly (Figures 4.33 and 4.34).

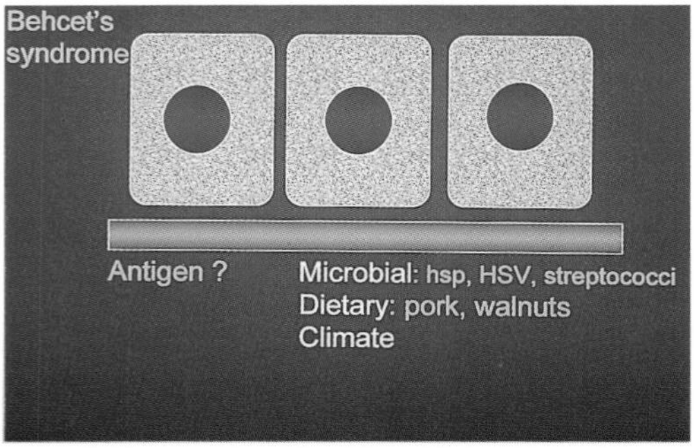

Figure 4.29
Behçet's syndrome: an immunological reaction to unknown antigens (hsp – heat shock protein; HSV – herpes simplex virus)

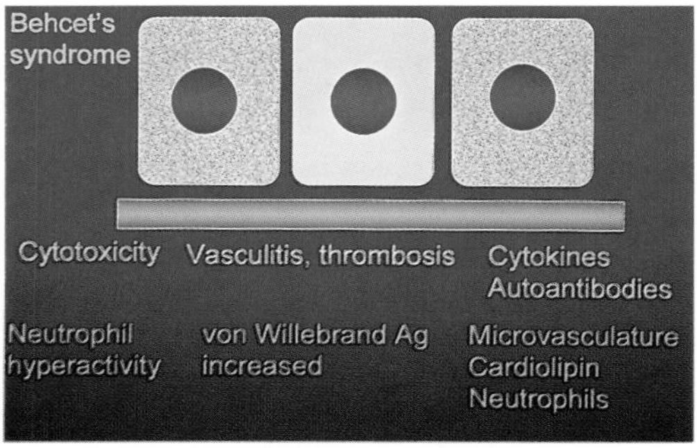

Figure 4.30
Behçet's syndrome: pathogenesis with neutrophil hyperactivity increases in autoantibodies to cardiolipin, neutrophils and microvasculature

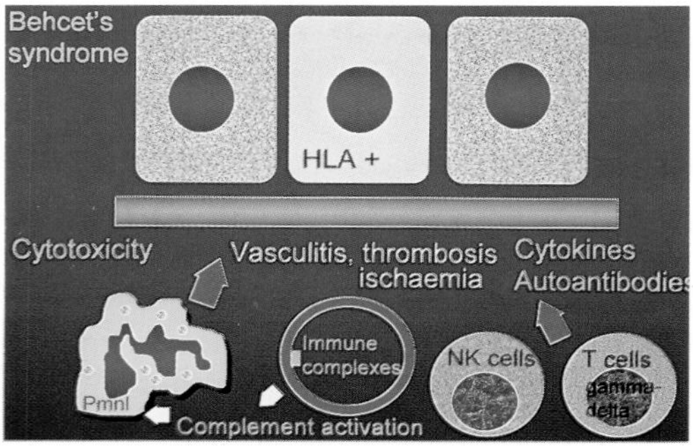

Figure 4.31
Behçet's syndrome: pathogenesis includes vasculitis and thrombosis

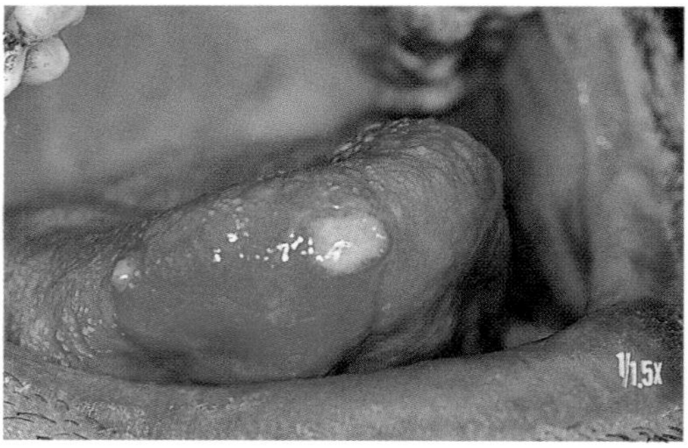

Figure 4.32
Behçet's syndrome typically causes oral ulceration

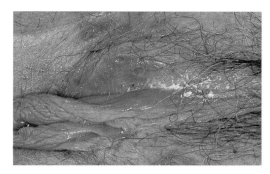

Figure 4.33
Behçet's syndrome:
vulval ulceration

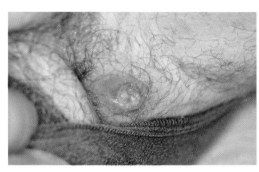

Figure 4.34
Behçet's syndrome:
perineal ulceration

Eyes: Visual acuity is often impaired. Uveitis (posterior uveitis: retinal vasculitis) is one of the more important ocular lesions and is more common in males.

Skin: Rashes include:

- An acneiform pustular rash;
- Pseudofolliculitis;
- Patients may develop pustules at the site of venepuncture (pathergy);
- Erythema nodosum (tender red nodules over the shins), particularly in females.

Neurological: Headache, psychiatric, motor or sensory manifestations.

Venous thrombosis: Thrombosis of large veins such as the vena cavae or dural sinuses may be caused by raised von Willebrand's factor, and can be life-threatening.

Joints: arthropathy of large joints such as the knees is not uncommon. Large joint arthropathy is not uncommon in Behçet's syndrome, but an overlap syndrome with relapsing polychondritis has also been described (mouth and genital ulcers with inflamed cartilage (MAGIC) syndrome).

Diagnosis

Other causes of this constellation of lesions, such as drugs, ulcerative colitis, Crohn's disease, mixed connective tissue disease, lupus erythematosus and Reiter's syndrome, should be excluded.

Diagnostic criteria for Behçet's syndrome are not completely agreed but include:

• Recurrent oral ulceration (more than 2 episodes in 12 months).

Plus two or more of the following:

• Recurrent genital ulceration;
• Eye lesions;
• Skin lesions;
• Pathergy.

There are no diagnostic laboratory criteria, but suggestive are:

• Pathergy;
• HLA B5101;
• Autoantibodies to cardiolipin, neutrophil cytoplasm, endothelium, phospholipids.

Management

Oral ulcers: treat as for aphthae (Tables 10.1, 10.2 and 10.5).
Systemic manifestations: may require aspirin, anticoagulants and immunosuppression using colchicine, corticosteroids, azathioprine, cyclosporin, dapsone, pentoxifylline, tacrolimus or thalidomide (Tables 4.6 and 10.7).

Table 4.6   Behçet's syndrome: therapy apart from corticosteroids

Lesions mainly	Drugs especially effective
Mouth ulcers	Thalidomide
Eye disease	Cyclosporin, azathioprine, tacrolimus, chlorambucil
Skin disease	Cyclosporin

Blastomycosis

Definition

A deep mycosis caused by *Blastomyces dermatitidis*

Incidence

Uncommon. North American blastomycosis is seen predominantly in the USA, in the Mississippi, Missouri and Ohio River valleys, and in Southern Canada, but also in Africa, India, the Middle East and Australia.

Age mainly affected

Adults

Sex mainly affected

M=F

Aetiology

Blastomyces dermatitidis found in soil and spores may be inhaled to produce respiratory and sometimes disseminated disease. Outdoor workers are particularly affected by blastomycosis, but it is increasingly seen in HIV disease.

Clinical features

Blastomycosis may produce ulcerating oral lesions.

Diagnosis

- Smear or culture;
- Biopsy;
- Skin tests and serology are unreliable.

Management

Ketoconazole, amphotericin, miconazole or itraconazole (Table 10.8).

Body art

Tattooing of the lip or other oral soft tissues, jewellry or art involving the teeth may occasionally be seen. Tattooing of the chin is seen increasingly in Maoris ('Moki') and may now be seen inside the lip in

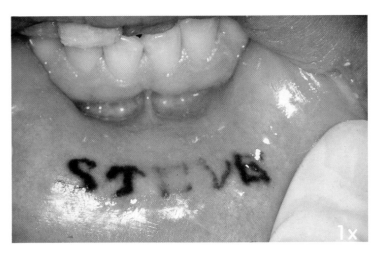

Figure 4.35
Body art: a tattoo in the labial mucosa

developed countries (Figure 4.35). The practice of piercing the oral and facial soft tissues and then placing foreign objects in the defects on a more or less permanent basis is one which has also been largely confined until recently to certain tribal groups in continental Africa and isolated Amazon regions of South America, for example, but it is now not uncommon in developed countries. Infections occasionally ensue.

Burning mouth

See Chapter 3

Burns

Burns are most commonly caused by:

- Heat on the palate or tongue mainly after the ingestion of hot foods or from reverse smoking;
- Ultraviolet light on the lower lip (actinic cheilitis) mainly in persons spending considerable time in the sun, such as skiers, windsurfers, fishermen, etc. (Figures 4.36 and 7.4);
- Ionizing radiation in the buccal or lingual mucosa (radiation mucositis);

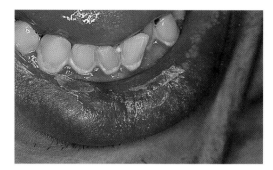

Figure 4.36
Actinic burn (Actinic cheilitis)

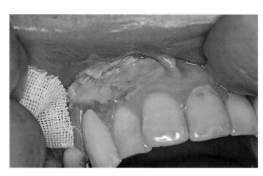

Figure 4.37
Chemical burn from topical aspirin

- Chemicals or drugs (Figure 4.37). Some patients attempt to relieve oral pain by holding an analgesic tablet at the site of pain. Aspirin commonly produces such burns. Mouthwashes, or the accidental ingestion of corrosive fluids may cause similar but more widespread lesions. Cytotoxic drugs often produce mucositis. Very rarely, burns are caused by illicit drugs or natural products such as the houseplant dieffenbachia, or the enzyme bromelin in pineapple;
- Cold uncommonly, but following cryosurgery;
- Electricity uncommonly, and seen usually in preschool children who bite electric flex.

Clinical features

Burns often manifest initially as a white lesion, later with sloughing mucosa. Mucositis is typically erythematous with erosions and ulcers.

Management

The management is to stop exposure to the causative agent. The lesions are usually self-healing but supportive care such as improved oral hygiene, chlorhexidine rinses and the use of a topical anti-inflammatory agent such as benzydamine often helps (Tables 10.1 and 10.2).

Cancrum oris (noma)

Definition

Gangrenous stomatitis

Incidence

Rare in the developed world

Age mainly affected

Children

Sex mainly affected

M=F

Aetiology

Acute necrotizing ulcerative gingivitis (ANUG) in malnourished, debilitated or severely immunocompromised patients may extend onto the oral mucosa and skin, resulting in cancrum oris. Anaerobes, particularly bacteroides species, treponemes and *Fusobacterium necrophorum* have been implicated.

Clinical features

Spreading necrosis eventually penetrates the buccal mucosa, leading to gangrene and ultimately a defect (orocutaneous fistula) and scarring.

Diagnosis

Clinical: an immune defect should always be excluded.

Management

- Local debridement and hygiene (Table 10.1);
- Improve nutrition;
- Systemic antibiotics;
- Plastic surgery as required.

Candidiasis (candidosis)

Thrush (acute pseudomembranous candidiasis)

Definition

This is a term used for the multiple white fleck appearance of acute candidiasis which purportedly resembles the appearance of the bird of the same name (Figure 4.38).

Incidence

Thrush is uncommon and is rare in healthy patients.

Age mainly affected

Adults

Sex mainly affected

M=F

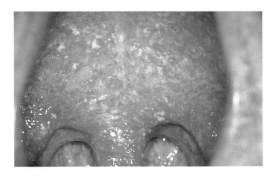

Figure 4.38
Thrush after use of a corticosteroid inhaler

Aetiology

Candida albicans is a harmless commensal in the mouths of nearly 50% of the population but, under suitable circumstances such as a disturbance in the oral flora or a decrease in immune defences, it can become an *opportunistic* pathogen. Thrush may be seen in healthy neonates however, or where the oral microflora is disturbed by antibiotics, corticosteroids or xerostomia. Oropharyngeal thrush occasionally complicates the use of steroid inhalers (Figures 4.38 and 4.39).

Thrush is often caused by immune defects, especially HIV infection, immunosuppressive treatment, leukaemias and lymphomas, cancer and diabetes. Infection is increasingly seen, mainly because of HIV infection, and now there is an increase both in nonalbicans species of *Candida* and resistance to antifungals. Candidiasis is an AIDS-defining condition.

Clinical features

Thrush presents mostly in the upper buccal vestibule posteriorly and the palate as white or creamy plaques (Figures 4.40–4.42)

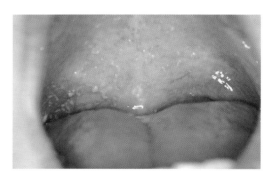

Figure 4.39
Thrush

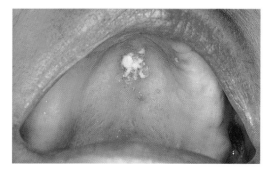

Figure 4.40
Thrush

that can be wiped off to leave a red base (Figure 4.42). Lesions may thus be white, or mixed white and red, and sometimes cause soreness.

Diagnosis

The diagnosis is usually clinical but a Gram-stained smear (hyphae) or oral rinse may help. Differentiation from lichen planus is the main problem (Figures 4.43 and 4.44) although occasionally hairy leukoplakia, leukoplakia, Koplik's or Fordyce's spots cause confusion.

Management

- Treat any predisposing cause and reduce smoking;
- Antifungals such as nystatin oral suspension, pastilles, amphotericin lozenges, miconazole gel or tablets, or fluconazole tablets (Table 10.8).

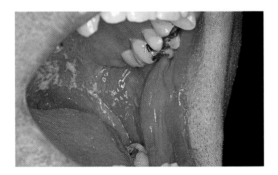

Figure 4.41
Thrush

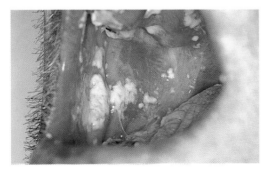

Figure 4.42
Thrush: in AIDS

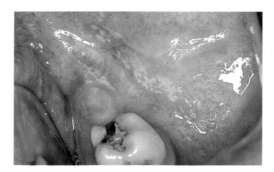

Figure 4.43
Thrush

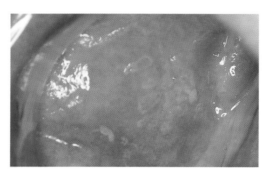

Figure 4.44
Thrush with bizarre configurations resembling lichen planus

Erythematous candidiasis

Definition
Red persistent lesions of candidiasis

Incidence
Uncommon

Age mainly affected
Adults

Sex mainly affected
M=F

Aetiology
Broad spectrum antimicrobials, xerostomia, smoking and HIV disease predispose.

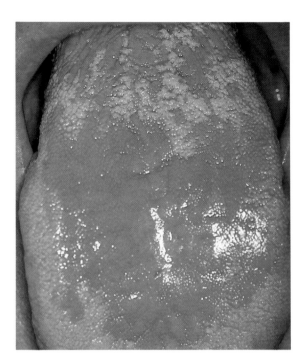

Figure 4.45
Erythematous candidiasis

Clinical features

Candidiasis may cause sore red mouth, especially of the tongue in patients on broad-spectrum antimicrobials (Figure 4.45). Erythematous candidiasis, especially on the palate or tongue, may also be a

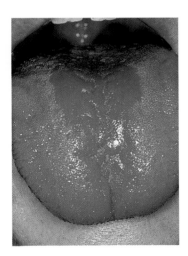

Figure 4.46
Erythematous candidiasis

feature of HIV disease. Median rhomboid glossitis is a red patch occurring in the middle of the dorsum in the posterior area of the anterior two-thirds of tongue (Figure 4.46) found especially in smokers.

Diagnosis

The diagnosis is usually clinical, but a Gram-stained smear (hyphae) or oral rinse may help.

Management

- Treat any predisposing cause;
- Antifungals such as nystatin oral suspension, pastilles, amphotericin lozenges, miconazole gel, tablets or fluconazole tablets (Table 10.8).

Chronic atrophic candidiasis (denture-induced stomatitis)

Chronic atrophic candidiasis is a candidal infection of the denture and denture-bearing mucosa (see Figure 4.47). Further detail is available on page 346.

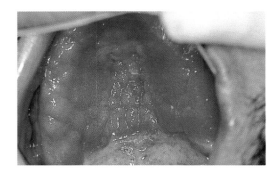

Figure 4.47
Chronic atrophic candidiasis is typically found beneath an upper denture (denture-induced stomatitis)

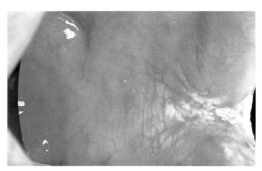

Figure 4.48
Chronic hyperplastic candidiasis in a typical location

Glossitis due to candidiasis

See Chapter 9

Chronic hyperplastic candidiasis

Candida may be associated with leukoplakia, especially at the commissures (page 157, Figures 4.48 and 4.109).

Chronic mucocutaneous candidiasis

Definition

Chronic mucocutaneous candidiasis is the term given to a number of rare syndromes characterized by persistent candidiasis affecting the mouth, skin, nails and other areas, due usually to a genetically determined immune defect mainly of T cells.

Incidence

Rare

Age mainly affected

From early childhood

Sex mainly affected

M=F

Aetiology

Congenital cellular immune defects of various types, sometimes poorly defined

Clinical features

Chronic mucocutaneous candidiasis (CMC) is a heterogeneous group of syndromes characterized by cutaneous, oral and other mucosal candidiasis, usually from early life. CMC presents with the following (Table 4.7).

Table 4.7   Types of chronic mucocutaneous candidiasis

CMC Type	Oral candidiasis	Other lesions
Localized	+	Oesophageal candidiasis
Diffuse	+	Candidal infection of oesophagus, pharynx, larynx and eyelids
Candidiasis–endocrinopathy	+	Hypoparathyroidism, hypoadrenocorticism, diabetes, pernicious anaemia, hypothyroidism and other autoimmune disorders
CMC with thymoma	+	Hypoimmunoglobulinaemia, myasthenia gravis

- Oral white plaques which eventually become widespread, thick and adherent (Figure 4.49) and the tongue fissured (Figure 4.50);
- Candidiasis involving both the skin and nails in varying severity (Figure 4.51);
- In one variant, candidiasis–endocrinopathy syndrome, hypoparathyroidism, dental defects and often hypoadrenocorticism, hypothyroidism and diabetes mellitus.

Diagnosis

- Clinical features;
- Immunological testing;
- Endocrinological testing.

Management

Systemic antifungals, especially fluconazole (Table 10.8). Patients should be followed up regularly, as there may be a predisposition to oral carcinoma.

Carcinoma

Definition

Malignant neoplasm of stratified squamous epithelium

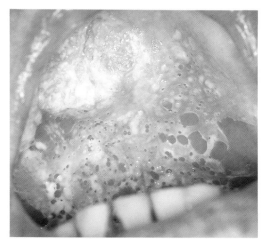

Figure 4.49
Chronic mucocutaneous candidiasis

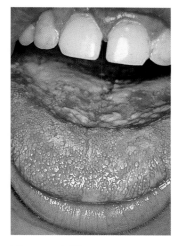

Figure 4.50
Chronic mucocutaneous candidiasis: persistent white lesions

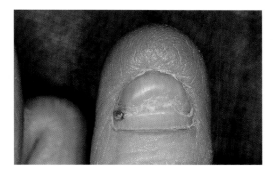

Figure 4.51
Chronic mucocutaneous candidiasis affecting nails

Incidence

Oral squamous cell carcinoma is uncommon in the developed world except in areas such as parts of France, but common in parts of the developing world such as South-East Asia, Brazil and Puerto Rico.

Age mainly affected

Middle-aged and elderly

Sex mainly affected

M>F

Aetiology

Aetiological factors acting on a genetically susceptible host who may have impaired metabolism of carcinogens, include:

- Tobacco use (75% smoke);
- Alcoholic beverages;
- Betel use;
- Diet poor in fresh fruit and vegetables;
- Infective agents (Candida, viruses).

In the case of lip carcinoma:

- Exposure to sunlight.

Second primary neoplasms are seen in up to 25% over 3 years, and in up to 40% of those who continue to smoke.

Potentially malignant oral lesions or conditions include:

- Dysplastic leukoplakias;
- Lichen planus;
- Oral submucous fibrosis;
- Chronic immunosuppression (lip cancer mainly).

Rare conditions such as:

- Tertiary syphilis;
- Discoid lupus erythematosus;
- Dyskeratosis congenita;
- Paterson–Kelly syndrome (sideropenic dysphagia).

Potentially malignant oral lesions frequently show epithelial atrophy and hence appear clinically particularly as red lesions, or erythroplasia. These are rare, isolated lesions or they may be associated with white lesions as erythroleukoplakia. The majority of erythroplasias show severe epithelial dysplasia or carcinoma in situ histologically. Other potentially malignant oral lesions may be associated with epithelial thickening and appear clinically as white lesions— leukoplakias—though this term is usually now restricted to those white lesions where no defined cause can be identified (see page 166). Leukoplakia is more common than erythroplasia.

Clinical features

A carcinoma can present as (Figures 4.52–4.55):

- Ulceration;
- Red lesion;

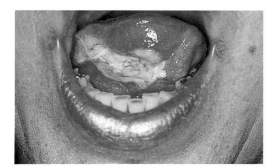

Figure 4.52
Carcinoma

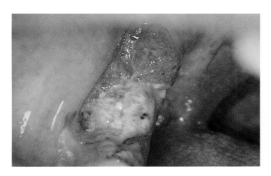

Figure 4.53
*Carcinoma of the
alveolus*

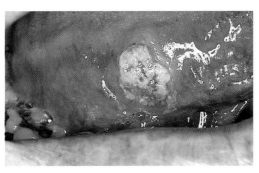

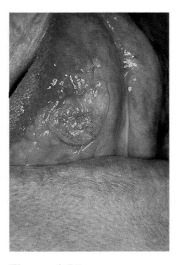

Figure 4.54
Carcinoma of the tongue

Figure 4.55
Carcinoma of the tongue

- White lesion;
- Lump;
- Fissure.

Carcinoma usually forms an indurated lump or solitary indurated
ulcer, with raised rolled edge and granular floor (Figure 4.56).
Cervical lymph node enlargement may be detectable (Figure 4.57).

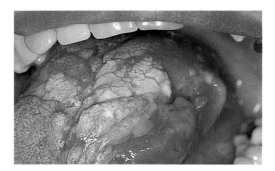

Figure 4.56
*Carcinoma in a typical
site on the posterolateral
border of the tongue*

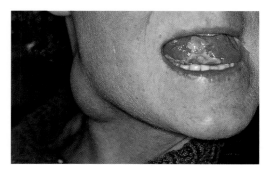

Figure 4.57
*Carcinoma with lymph
node metastasis*

Intraorally, carcinoma typically affects the posterolateral tongue, with submandibular lymph node involvement (Figure 4.57). Lip carcinoma presents with thickening, induration, crusting or ulceration, usually at vermilion border of the lower lip just to one side of the midline. There is late involvement of the submental lymph nodes (Chapter 7).

Diagnosis

Almost invariably indicated are biopsy and specialist referral. It is essential to differentiate an intraoral carcinoma from other causes of mouth ulcers, especially major aphthae or, rarely, chronic infections (e.g. tuberculosis or mycoses). A lip carcinoma must be differentiated mainly from herpes labialis, keratoacanthoma and basal cell carcinoma. It is crucial to determine whether cervical lymph nodes are involved or if there are other primary tumours or metastases elsewhere, particularly in the upper aerodigestive tract (pharynx, larynx, oesophagus, bronchi).

Variants

Most carcinomas are squamous cell carcinomas, but variants include the following:

- Verrucous carcinoma: a superficial exophytic well-differentiated non-metastasizing lesion mainly seen in elderly males, amenable to excision with a good prognosis;
- Spindle cell carcinoma: a rare poorly differentiated carcinoma seen mainly in the lip or tongue, with an aggressive course. It is usually treated surgically;
- Adenosquamous carcinoma: a rare aggressive carcinoma usually affecting the floor of mouth or palate and having considerable metastatic potential and a poor prognosis;
- Adenoid squamous carcinoma: a low-grade malignant neoplasm seen mainly on the lower lip and very amenable to excision;
- Basaloid squamous carcinoma: an aggressive neoplasm seen mainly in the base of tongue or fauces in males, metastasizing widely.

Management

The prognosis of squamous cell carcinoma is better with early detection but is very site dependent. Oral carcinoma is usually staged using the Tumour, Node, Metastasis (TNM) system (Tables 4.8 and 4.9). It is now treated by surgery and/or irradiation. Occasionally, chemotherapy is used but is rarely of significant value.

Synchronous and metachronous primary tumours elsewhere in the oral cavity or in the upper aerodigestive tract must be excluded by radiography, endoscopy and biopsy. The prognosis for:

- Intraoral carcinoma is as low as about a 30% 5-year survival rate because of the high proportion of late-stage cases;

Table 4.8   TMN system

Stage	T=primary tumour	N=regional lymph nodes	M=metastases at a distance
0	No evidence	No palpable node	None detectable
1is	Ca in situ	No palpable node	None detectable
1	Tumour <2 cm	Suspicious palpable ipsilateral node	Clinical or radiological evidence of metastasis
2	2–4 cm	Suspicious palpable contralateral or bilateral node	—
3	>4 cm	Palpable large fixed node	—
4	Tumour invades adjacent structures	—	—

Table 4.9 TNM clinical staging and prognosis of intraoral cancer

Stage	T	N	M	5-year survival (%)
1	1	0	0	85
2	2	0	0	65
3	3	0	0	40
	1	1	0	
	2	1	0	
	3	1	0	
4	1	2 or 3	0	10
	2	2 or 3	0	
	3	2 or 3	0	
	Any	Any	1	

- Lip carcinoma, typically detected at an earlier stage, is much better, often more than a 70% 5-year survival.

Aftercare

Predisposing factors such as tobacco and alcohol use should be stopped; patients are liable to subsequent further primary tumours, especially in the mouth and respiratory tract.

Radiation-induced lesions are invariable if teletherapy (external beam) involves the oral mucosa and salivary glands. The consequences may include the following:

Mucositis: diffuse erythema and ulceration (Figures 4.58 and 4.143).

Xerostomia: leading to:

- Dysphagia;
- Disturbed taste;
- Radiation caries;

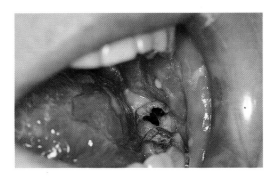

Figure 4.58
Radiation mucositis

- Candidiasis;
- Sialadenitis.

Liability to osteoradionecrosis;
Trismus;
Telangiectasia;
In children:

- Jaw hypoplasia;
- Hypoplasia and retarded eruption of developing teeth.

Biopsy, surgery and tooth extraction should be avoided wherever possible. Treatment is mainly symptomatic with control of infections. Treatment with antimicrobials active against Gram-negative bacilli may help reduce or prevent mucositis. Xerostomia is managed as discussed elsewhere (see Chapters 1 and 5).

Cat scratch disease

Definition

Lymphadenopathy and fever following a cat scratch

Incidence

Uncommonly reported

Age mainly affected

Children

Sex mainly affected

M=F

Aetiology

Rochalimaea (Bartonella) quintana, a small pleomorphic bacillus transmitted by cats, usually by a scratch

Clinical features

Three to 5 days after contact there is a papule which vesiculates and then heals. There may be fever and there is always tender regional lymphadenitis. Sometimes there is a rash or other complications.

Diagnosis

The diagnosis is clinical.

Management

Erythromycin

Cheek chewing (morsicatio buccarum)

Cheek or lip biting is often a neurotic trait. The mucosa is shredded with a shaggy white appearance similar to that of white sponge naevus (page 234) but restricted to areas close to the occlusal line (Figures 4.59 and 4.107).

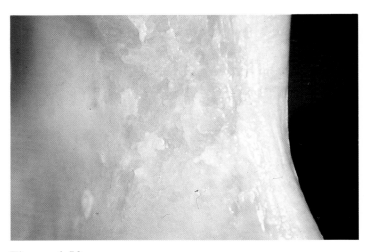

Figure 4.59
Cheek biting

Chemotherapy-induced lesions

There are immediate ulcerative, haemorrhagic and infective oral complications of chemotherapy which resolve once treatment is finished. Chemotherapy may however have long-term effects on salivary function, and on hard tissues that were developing at the time, including the teeth that were mineralizing when treatment was given which may show crown abnormalities (hypoplasia, microdontia or taurodontism) and root anomalies (shortened, constricted, tapered or thinned) or the teeth may fail to develop. Facial growth is also disturbed.

Chickenpox

Definition

A rash caused by varicella-zoster virus infection which goes through macular, papular, vesicular and pustular stages, concentrated mainly on the trunk and head and neck.

Incidence

This is a common infection seen mainly in epidemics.

Age mainly affected

Children

Sex mainly affected

M=F

Aetiology

Varicella (chickenpox) is a highly contagious airborne infection caused by the varicella-zoster virus (VZV). After primary infection, which may be subclinical, VZV remains latent in dorsal root ganglia, including the trigeminal ganglion in some patients. Reactivation of the VZV may result in herpes zoster (shingles).

Clinical features

After an incubation period of 2–3 weeks, primary clinical infection may present with chickenpox:

- Fever;
- Malaise, irritability, anorexia;
- Rash variably dense, concentrated mainly on the trunk and head and neck (i.e. centripetal). The rash crops in waves over 2–4 days, so that lesions at different stages are typically seen. The typical rash goes through macular, papular, vesicular and pustular stages before crusting.

The oral lesions include:

- Vesicles, especially in the palate, which rupture to produce ulcers;
- Ulcers, painful, round or ovoid with an inflammatory halo (Figure 4.60);
- Cervical lymphadenitis.

Diagnosis

Diagnosis of chickenpox is usually on clinical grounds. Viral culture, immunostaining or electron microscopy are indicated mainly in immunocompromised patients. A rising serum antibody titre is confirmatory.

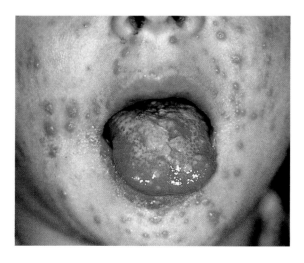

Figure 4.60
Chickenpox showing rash and mouth ulcers

Management

Treatment is symptomatic; immune globulin or aciclovir may be indicated in immunocompromised patients. Valaciclovir or famciclovir may be needed for aciclovir-resistant VZV infections.

Chronic ulcerative stomatitis

In this rare chronic ulcerative condition which mimics lichen planus, antinuclear antibodies against stratified squamous epithelium are seen as a speckled pattern in the basal and parabasal layers. IgG is deposited, with fibrin at the basement membrane zone. Hydroxychloroquine appears to be effective treatment.

Coccidioidomycosis

Definition

A deep mycosis caused by *Coccidioides immitis*

Incidence

Rare. Seen mainly in arid areas such as South-West USA, Mexico, Central America and parts of South America

Age mainly affected

Adults

Sex mainly affected

M=F

Aetiology

Inhalation of spores, found in soil, produces subclinical infection in up to 90% of the population in endemic areas. Pregnant women, Blacks, Philippinos, Mexicans and immunocompromised persons are prone to disseminated coccidioidomycosis.

Clinical features

Clinical illness presents typically as:

- Acute pulmonary disease;
- Fever (San Joaquin valley fever);
- Sometimes erythema nodosum or erythema multiforme;
- Rare verrucous oral lesions, sometimes with infection of the jaw, typically secondary to lung involvement.

Diagnosis

- Biopsy;
- Serology;
- Spherulin or coccidioidin skin tests

Management

Systemic amphotericin, sometimes supplemented with ketoconazole, itraconazole or fluconazole (Table 10.8)

Coeliac disease (gluten-sensitive enteropathy)

Definition

Hypersensitivity to gluten, a constituent of wheat and other cereals

Incidence

Uncommon, but coeliac disease is not uncommon in some ethnic groups such as celtic descendants; although not always recognized if not severe.

Age mainly affected

From childhood

Sex mainly affected

M=F

Aetiology

Coeliac disease is a genetically determined hypersensitivity to gluten that affects the jejunum, leading to antibodies against endomysium and gliadin, malabsorption and predisposing to lymphomas.

Clinical features

Patients may appear otherwise well; a few fail to thrive and/or have other manifestations of malabsorption. A small percentage of patients with aphthae have coeliac disease causing malabsorption and deficiencies of haematinics, resulting in oral ulceration. Oral features of coeliac disease may include:

- Ulcers (Figure 4.61) and occasionally dermatitis herpetiformis (page 121);
- Angular stomatitis;
- Glossitis or burning mouth syndrome;
- Dental hypoplasia.

Diagnosis

A blood picture and haematinic assay may suggest malabsorption but small bowel biopsy and autoantibodies are required for definitive diagnosis.

Management

Deficiencies should be rectified and the patient must thereafter adhere to a gluten-free diet. The oral lesions then invariably ameliorate.

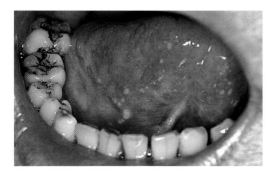

Figure 4.61
Coeliac disease manifesting with aphthae

Congenital immunodeficiencies

Chronic oral candidiasis, which may present as thrush and/or angular stomatitis, is an early and prominent feature in cell-mediated (T cell) immune defects, and there is a predisposition to recurrent lesions of herpes simplex and varicella-zoster virus. There are many primary immune defects known, some barely compatible with life. They include the following:

- Selective IgA deficiency. This is the most common immunoglobulin deficiency and the main primary (genetically determined) immune defect. Some patients are healthy, but others, particularly those who also lack IgG_2, suffer recurrent respiratory infection, autoimmune disorders and atopy. Many have mouth ulcers, and there may be a reduced protection against dental caries;
- Di George syndrome. This branchial arch defect affects the thymus and has additional profound defects such as cardiovascular defects and hypoparathyroidism;
- Wiskott–Aldrich syndrome. A rare immune deficiency syndrome with thrombocytopenia and eczema, it is associated with oral petechiae, oral ulceration, premature tooth loss and/or large pulp chambers;
- Chronic granulomatous disease (CGD) affects males mainly. Neutrophils and monocytes are defective at killing catalase-positive micro-organisms such as staphylococci. It presents typically with cervical lymph node enlargement and suppuration, and recurrent infections from early childhood which may result in enamel hypoplasia. There is also a predisposition to mouth ulcers and periodontal destruction;
- Sex-linked panhypoimmunoglobulinaemia (Bruton's syndrome) affects males almost exclusively and presents mainly with recurrent pyogenic respiratory infections and mouth ulcers.

Cowden's syndrome (multiple hamartoma and neoplasia syndrome)

Definition

This is an autosomal dominant condition of multiple hamartomas.

Incidence

Rare; mainly seen in Caucasians

Age mainly affected

From birth

Sex mainly affected

M=F

Aetiology

Autosomal dominant

Clinical features

- Papillomatous lesions and tricholemmomas on the skin especially over the neck, nose and ear;
- Oral lesions; papules, fissured tongue, hypoplasia of the uvula, and maxillary and mandibular hypoplasia;
- Malignant disease, particularly carcinomas of breast, thyroid and colon. These typically are preceded by the oral lesions;
- Uterine leiomyomas;
- Keratoses on the palms and soles; learning disability and motor incoordination.

Diagnosis

This is clinical mainly, supported by lesional biopsies.

Management

The patient should be closely followed in order to detect any malignancy at an early stage.

Crohn's disease

Definition

Crohn's disease is a chronic inflammatory bowel disease of unknown aetiology, affecting mainly the ileum (regional ileitis).

Incidence

Uncommon

Age mainly affected

From early adulthood; usually 2nd and 3rd decades

Sex mainly affected

M>F

Aetiology

Idiopathic; some have a postulated reaction to food or other antigens such as paratuberculosis.

Clinical features

- Chronic inflammatory bowel disease, affecting mainly the ileum and presenting typically with abdominal pain, persistent diarrhoea with passage of blood and mucus, anaemia and weight loss. However, any part of the gastrointestinal tract can be involved, including the mouth;
- Oral lesions are most likely in those who develop skin, eye or joint complications and include:
  - Swelling of the lips (Figure 4.62);
  - Angular stomatitis;
  - Persistent irregular oral ulcers or classic aphthae (Figure 4.63);
  - Gingival swelling;
  - Mucosal tags (Figure 4.64);

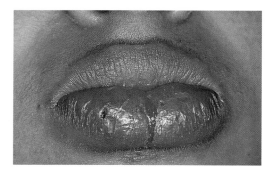

Figure 4.62
Crohn's disease presenting with labial swelling and fissuring

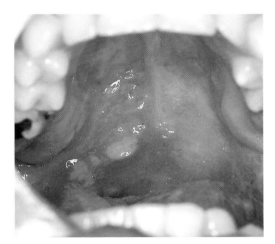

Figure 4.63
Crohn's disease:
ulceration

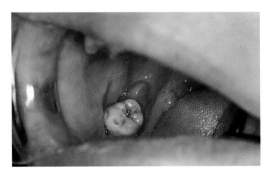

Figure 4.64
Crohn's disease: mucosal
tags in a common site

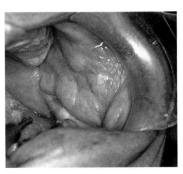

Figure 4.65
Crohn's disease:
'cobblestoning' of
mucosa

- Folding of the oral mucosa may lead to a 'cobblestone' appearance (Figure 4.65).
- Melkersson–Rosenthal syndrome, a related condition, is discussed on page189;
- Orofacial granulomatosis, a related condition, is discussed on page 198.

Diagnosis

- An oral biopsy may confirm the presence of lymphoedema and granulomas;
- Blood tests for full blood picture, and levels of albumin, calcium, folate, iron and vitamin B12;
- Intestinal radiology, endoscopy, and biopsy to detect bowel involvement. Radiolabelled leukocyte studies may help.

Management

- Secondary nutritional deficiencies should be corrected;
- Intralesional corticosteroids may help control oral lesions such as swelling;
- Systemic sulphasalazine or other agents may be indicated.

Cryptococcosis

Definition

A deep mycosis caused by *Cryptococcus neoformans*

Incidence

Uncommon

Age mainly affected

Adults

Sex mainly affected

M=F

Aetiology

Cryptococcosis is seen worldwide from aspiration of spores found in excreta from pigeons, canaries, parrots and budgerigars, and in rotting fruit and vegetables.

Clinical features

In healthy persons, infection is typically subclinical. In immunocompromised persons there may be:

- Cryptococcal meningoencephalitis; untreated this is fatal in over 70%;
- Dissemination to the meninges, heart, spleen, pancreas, adrenals, ovaries, muscles, bones, liver and gastrointestinal tract;
- Oral nonhealing extraction wounds, or chronic ulcers on the palate or tongue.

Diagnosis

- Biopsy;
- Smear.;
- Culture;
- Assay of serum or CSF for capsular antigen and antibody (latex agglutination test).

Management

Amphotericin, ketoconazole, fluconazole or itraconazole (Table 10.8)

Cyclic neutropenia

This is a rare condition (Figure 4.66) which may respond to granulo-cyte colony stimulating factor (GCSF), and characterized by:

- Cyclical fall in neutrophil counts every 21 days;
- Recurrent pyogenic infections;
- Recurrent mouth ulcers;
- Advanced periodontitis.

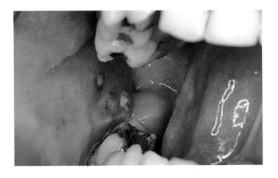

Figure 4.66
Cyclic neutropenia presenting with recurring mouth ulcers

Darier's disease

This rare inherited skin disease (keratosis follicularis) can occasionally involve the mouth, especially the palate, with white plaques or papules resembling stomatitis nicotina. Oral lesions are seen only where there is cutaneous involvement and they may sometimes constrict salivary ducts.

Denture-induced hyperplasia (denture granuloma; epulis fissuratum)

Definition

Hyperplasia related to a denture flange

Incidence

Common

Age mainly affected

Middle-aged or elderly patients

Sex mainly affected

M=F

Aetiology

Where a denture flange irritates the vestibular mucosa, an ulcer (Figure 4.67) and then a linear reparative process may be initiated. In time, an elongated fibroepithelial enlargement may develop (Figure 4.68). Such a lesion (a denture granuloma) differs little in structure from a fibroepithelial polyp and is not a granuloma.

Clinical features

It is usually related to a lower complete denture, especially anteriorly. Typically seen in patients wearing ill-fitting dentures, there is a painless lump with a smooth pink surface lying parallel to the alveolar ridge and sometimes grooved by the denture flange. Several leaflets with a fairly firm consistency may develop.

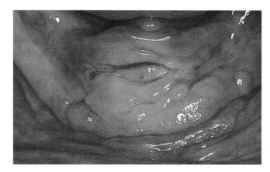

Figure 4.67
*Denture-induced
ulceration and
hyperplasia*

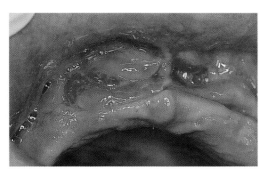

Figure 4.68
*Denture-induced
hyperplasia*

Diagnosis

This is initially a clinical diagnosis.

Management

Relieve the denture flange. Although rarely symptomatic, a denture granuloma should be excised and examined histologically if modification of the denture does not induce the lesion to regress within 2–3 weeks. Rarely, a denture granuloma arises because a lesion, e.g. antral carcinoma, develops beneath a denture and rubs on it.

Dermatitis herpetiformis

Definition

Dermatitis herpetiformis is a rare skin disorder which is characterized by an itchy rash often over the shoulders, and is frequently associated with gluten sensitivity.

Incidence

Rare

Age mainly affected

Adult, second or third decades

Sex mainly affected

M>F

Aetiology

IgA-autoantibody-mediated local tissue damage and gluten sensitivity may be involved. There is an association with HLA-B8 and HLA-DR3 and antibodies as in a coeliac disease.

Clinical features

- An itchy rash on the extensor surfaces, particularly of the upper limbs;
- Oral lesions mainly affect the palate, buccal mucosa or gingiva, and usually follow skin lesions, although occasionally this sequence is reversed. Lesions may be:
  - Erythematous;
  - Purpuric;
  - Vesicular;
  - Ulcerative.
- Enamel hypoplasia may be seen;
- There is a small risk of gastrointestinal malignancy.

Diagnosis

- Biopsy of oral lesions with immunostaining is useful; granular IgA and C3 deposits are detectable at the tips of dermal papillae in lesional tissue, and in apparently normal oral mucosa in up to 45% of cases;
- Serology is of little diagnostic value although patients can have circulating antiendomysium antibodies.

Management

- Oral lesions tend to respond to systemic dapsone; sulphapyridine may be a useful alternative therapy;
- A gluten-free diet should be used, though it is unclear what effect this has on the course of oral lesions.

Drug-induced hyperpigmentation

A variety of drugs cause pigmentation rarely, and often by unknown mechanisms. In the past, heavy metals (e.g. lead) caused pigmented lines because of sulphide deposits in gingival pockets. Drugs currently implicated include antimalarials, busulphan, cisplatin, phenothiazines, ACTH, zidovudine, minocycline and oral contraceptives. Diagnosis is usually from a history of exposure to the drug.

Drug-induced ulcers

Aetiology

A wide spectrum of drugs can occasionally cause mouth lesions, by various mechanisms (Figure 4.69). Ulcers are common in those on cytotoxic drugs. Other reactions are uncommon or rare. The more common examples include the following:

- Cytotoxic agents, particularly methotrexate;
- Agents producing lichen-planus-like (lichenoid) lesions, such as antihypertensives, antidiabetics, gold salts, nonsteroidal anti-inflammatory agents, antimalarials and other drugs;

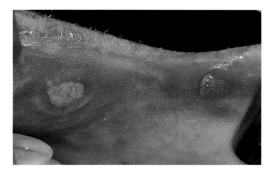

Figure 4.69
Drug-induced ulcers in leukaemia

- Agents causing local chemical burns (especially aspirin held in the mouth);
- Agents causing erythema multiforme (especially sulphonamides and barbiturates);
- Other drugs such as nicorandil and alendronate.

Clinical features

Cytotoxic-induced ulcers: these have a nonspecific appearance.
Lichenoid lesions: resemble lichen planus clinically and histologically (see page 169).
Chemical burns: are usually solitary lesions with sloughing of mucosa.
Erythema multiforme: ulcers and lip swelling (see Chapter 7).

Diagnosis

Diagnosis is made from the drug history and testing the effect of drug withdrawal. Skin patch tests are rarely of practical value.

Management

Treatment is to stop the causative drug and treat ulceration symptomatically with topical benzydamine and possibly chlorhexidine (Tables 10.1 and 10.2).

Dyskeratosis congenita (Zinser–Engman–Cole syndrome)

This is a rare autosomal dominant or X-linked disorder (most patients are male) characterized by the following:

- Oral blistering, ulceration, scarring and lichenoid white lesions; most have oral leukoplakia by the age of 5–10 years;
- Cutaneous grey-brown reticular hyperpigmentation;
- Pancytopenia and other lesions; telangiectasia, bullae and ectropion, hyperhidrosis, thin hair.

Oral verrucous leukoplakia or carcinoma can arise.

Ectopic sebaceous glands

In some people sebaceous glands may be seen as creamy-yellow dots (Fordyce spots) along the border between the vermilion and the oral mucosa (Figure 4.70). There are no associated hair follicles.

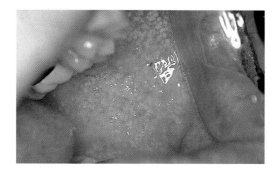

Figure 4.70
Fordyce spots: sebaceous glands in the buccal mucosa

Fordyce spots are not usually evident in infants, but they appear in children after the age of 3 years, increase during puberty and then again in later adult life. About 80–90% of adults have these spots.

No treatment is indicated or available.

Epidermolysis bullosa

Definition

Epidermolysis bullosa (EB) is a group of rare inherited disorders of skin and mucosa, mostly characterized by vesiculation at the epithelial basement membrane zone in response to minor trauma, and consequent scarring.

An acquired form of EB (epidermolysis bullosa acquisita) is a chronic blistering disease of skin and mucosae with autoantibodies to type VII procollagen of epithelial basement membranes.

Incidence

Rare

Age mainly affected

From early childhood

Sex mainly affected

M=F

Aetiology

Defect in epithelial basement membrane attachment due to a collagen VII defect.

Clinical features

- Bullae appear early in life in some subtypes, often precipitated by suckling;
- Blisters break down to persistent ulcers that eventually heal with scarring;
- The tongue becomes depapillated and scarred;
- Enamel hypoplasia may be seen in some subtypes;
- Oral hygiene tends to be neglected in view of the fragility of mucosa, with subsequent caries and periodontal disease;
- Squamous cell carcinoma is a rare complication.

Oral lesions are most common in the junctional types of EB, but rare in most nonscarring simplex types of epidermolysis bullosa, in which the vesiculation is intraepithelial. Scarring in the dystrophic form affects the extremities including the nails (Table 4.10).

Table 4.10

EB type	Oral lesions
Epidermolytic (simplex)	Mucosal lesions in some subtypes. Anodontia in Kallin subtype
Junctional	Mucosal lesions and enamel hypoplasia
Dermolytic (dystrophic)	Mucosal lesions and enamel hypoplasia in Hallopeau–Siemens subtypes

Diagnosis

Clinical features

Management

- Attention to oral hygiene and caries prevention;
- Attention to nutrition;
- Prevent trauma and infections;
- Phenytoin may help some forms.

Erythema multiforme

See Chapter 7

Erythroplasia (erythroplakia)

Definition

Erythroplasia (erythroplakia) is a rare condition defined as 'any lesion of the oral mucosa that presents as bright red velvety plaques which cannot be characterised clinically or pathologically as any other recognisable condition' (WHO, 1978).

Incidence

Rare

Age mainly affected

Elderly

Sex mainly affected

M>F

Aetiology

The aetiology is unclear.

Clinical features

Erythroplasia is:

- A velvety red plaque, usually level with or depressed below surrounding mucosa (Figure 4.71);
- Usually seen on the soft palate or ventrum of the tongue/floor of the mouth;
- Sometimes associated with white patches;
- Usually potentially malignant; there are areas of dysplasia, carcinoma in situ or invasive carcinoma in virtually every case of erythroplasia. Carcinomas are seen 17 times more frequently in erythroplakia than in leukoplakia and these are therefore the most potentially malignant of all oral mucosal lesions—but erythroplasia is far less common than leukoplakia and lichen planus.

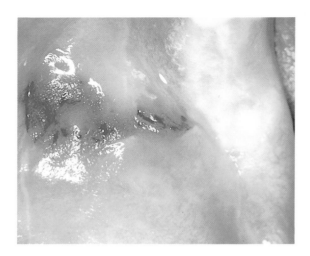

Figure 4.71
Erythroplasia

Diagnosis

Biopsy is indicated.

Management

Treatment is by excision but the prognosis is often poor.

Fibroma

Definition

Benign neoplasms arising from fibroblasts

Incidence

Rare

Age mainly affected

Adults

Sex mainly affected

M=F

Aetiology

A benign neoplasm of fibroblastic origin

Clinical features

Many lesions, called fibromas in the past, were fibroepithelial polyps. The true fibroma is a continuously enlarging new growth, not necessarily arising at a site of potential trauma. It is a pedunculated growth with smooth nonulcerated pink surface.

Diagnosis

Clinical supported by excision biopsy

Management

Removal should be total, deep and wide.

Fibroepithelial polyps

Definition

A localized tissue overgrowth that generally takes the form of a smooth, sessile or pedunculated polyp

Incidence

Common

Age mainly affected

Adults

Sex mainly affected

M=F

Aetiology

Fibrous lumps appear to be purely reparative in nature. When oral tissues are traumatized, healing is usually rapid and complete with negligible scar formation. Sometimes a more vigorous and extensive healing process ensues, producing a localized tissue overgrowth which generally takes the form of a smooth, sessile or pedunculated polyp.

Clinical features

The variable inflammatory changes account for the different clinical presentations of fibrous lumps from red, shiny and soft lumps to those which are pale, stippled and firm. Commonly they are round, painless pedunculated swellings arising from the marginal or papillary gingiva (epulides), and sometimes adjacent to sites of irritation (eg a carious cavity) (Figures 4.72–4.74). They may reach quite a large size, and may become ulcerated if traumatized.

Diagnosis

Diagnosis is clinical, supported by excision biopsy.

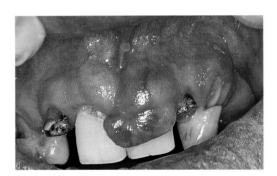

Figure 4.72
Fibrous lump (fibrous epulis)

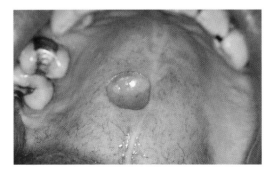

Figure 4.73
Fibrous lump

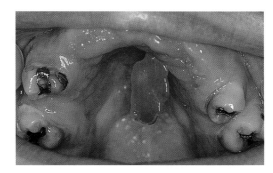

Figure 4.74
Fibrous lump
(fibroepithelial polyp)

Management

Fibrous lumps should be excised with their entire base and examined histologically.

Fibrous histiocytoma

This benign tumour arises usually in the 5th decade as a slow-growing and firm swelling, typically in the tongue, buccal mucosa, gingiva or lip. It should be excised.

Focal dermal hypoplasia (Goltz syndrome)

This is a rare X-linked syndrome characterized by:

- Skin atrophy, pigmentary changes and telangiectasia;
- Alopecia;
- Syndactyly or polydactyly;
- Strabismus or anophthalmia;
- Oral papillomatous lesions;
- Hypodontia.

Focal palmoplantar and oral hyperkeratosis syndrome

This is a rare autosomal dominant disorder characterized by oral white lesions and palmoplantar hyperkeratosis. Nail thickening and hyperhidrosis are not usually seen. Oral lesions typically affect gingivae, palate and lateral margins of the tongue.

Fordyce spots (ectopic sebaceous glands)

See page 124

Gluten-sensitive enteropathy

See coeliac disease, page 112

Haemangioma

Definition

A hamartoma of blood vessels producing reddish, bluish or purplish soft lesions which blanch on pressure

Incidence

Common

Age mainly affected

From childhood

Sex mainly affected

M=F

Aetiology

Haemangiomas are benign lesions of developmental origin—hamartomas.

Clinical features

Many haemangiomas appear in infancy, most by the age of 2 years. They grow slowly but, by the age of 10, the majority have involuted. Oral angiomas are seen most often on the tongue or lip, as painless reddish, bluish or purplish soft lesions (Figures 4.75–4.77). The characteristic feature is that they blanch on pressure, or contain blood on aspiration with a needle and syringe.

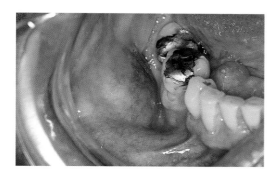

Figure 4.75
Haemangioma

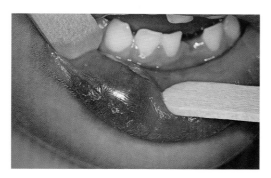

Figure 4.76
Haemangioma in the lip

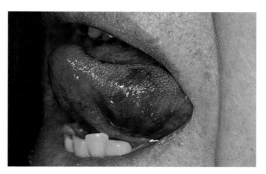

Figure 4.77
Haemangioma

Diagnosis

- Diagnosis is clinical;
- Aspiration for confirmation;
- Gadolinium scan occasionally.

Management

Some 50% of haemangiomas present in childhood regress spontaneously. Not all need treatment, but if they do for aesthetic or functional reasons, cryosurgery, laser surgery or injection of sclerosing agents are very effective. Very large haemangiomas may need to be treated with embolization, but only if bleeding is troublesome.

Hand, foot and mouth disease (vesicular stomatitis with exanthem)

Definition

Vesicles and ulcers in oropharynx, with vesicles on hands and/or feet, in small epidemics in children

Incidence

Uncommonly reported

Age mainly affected

In epidemics in children

Sex mainly affected

M=F

Aetiology

Coxsackie virus A16 is usually implicated, but A5, A7, A9 and A10 or viruses of the Coxsackie B9 group, or other enteroviruses (RNA), may be responsible. Infections may be subclinical.

Clinical features

The incubation period is up to a week. The infection produces the following:

- Skin vesicles that are small, painful and surrounded by inflammatory haloes, especially on the dorsum and lateral aspect of the fingers and toes (Figure 4.78). A rash is not always present or may affect more proximal parts of the limbs or buttocks;

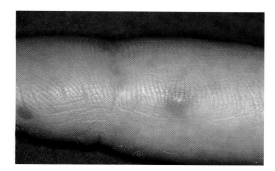

Figure 4.78
Hand foot and mouth disease

- Oral ulcers usually affect the tongue or buccal mucosa and are shallow, painful, very small and surrounded by inflammatory haloes (Figure 4.79) resembling herpetic stomatitis, but with no gingivitis and only mild fever, malaise and anorexia.

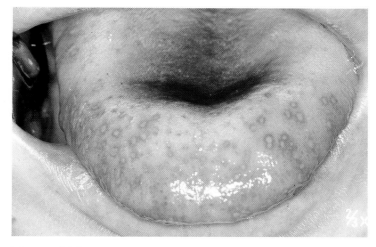

Figure 4.79
Hand foot and mouth disease

Diagnosis

This is a clinical diagnosis. Serology is confirmatory but rarely required.

Management

There is no specific treatment available. The skin vesicles usually heal spontaneously in about 1 week. The mouth lesions can be treated symptomatically (see Herpes simplex, page 139 and Tables 10.1, 10.2).

Hereditary benign intraepithelial dyskeratosis

This is a rare autosomal dominant defect in keratinization, seen mainly in the USA, that results in white lesions in the buccal and lingual mucosae, and plaques on the conjunctivae.

Hereditary haemorrhagic telangiectasia (HHT; Osler–Rendu–Weber syndrome)

Definition

Multiple inherited telangiectasia in mouth and upper respiratory and gastrointestinal tracts

Incidence

Rare

Age mainly affected

From puberty

Sex mainly affected

M=F

Aetiology

Autosomal dominant condition

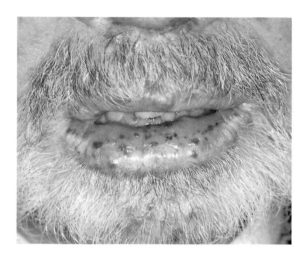

Figure 4.80
*Hereditary
haemorrhagic
telangiectasia: this
patient bled
repeatedly from his
mouth, becoming
profoundly anaemic*

Clinical features

Telangiectases are present:

- Orally (Figure 4.80);
- Periorally;
- Also in nose, gastrointestinal tract and occasionally on palms.

Telangiectases may bleed, resulting in iron-deficiency anaemia.

Diagnosis

- Clinical features;
- Blood picture;
- Differentiate from other causes of telangiectasia such as sclero-derma, chronic liver disease and postirradiation.

Management

Cryosurgery or laser if bleeding is troublesome; treat anaemia

Hereditary mucoepithelial dysplasia

This is a rare autosomal dominant condition characterized by:

- Red patches in the oral, pharyngeal, nasal, genital and conjunctival mucosae;

- Rough dry skin;
- Photophobia, nystagmus, corneal vascularization, cataracts and keratitis;
- Hair thinning or alopecia;
- Dry rough skin;
- Pneumonia, emphysema and lung fibrosis.

There is no known malignant potential.

Herpangina

Definition

Vesicles and ulcers in oropharynx, in small epidemics in children

Incidence

Uncommonly reported

Age mainly affected

Children

Sex mainly affected

M=F

Aetiology

Herpangina is usually caused by enteroviruses, mainly Coxsackie viruses A1–A6, A8, A10, A12, A16 or A22, but similar syndromes can be caused by other viruses, especially Coxsackie B (B1, 2, 3, 4 or 5) and echoviruses (9 or 17).

Clinical features

Herpangina presents with:

- Fever, malaise;
- Headache, and a sore throat caused by an ulcerating vesicular eruption in the oropharynx;

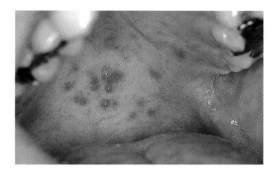

Figure 4.81
Herpangina: ulcers in the soft palate mainly

- Vesicles mainly on the fauces and soft palate, which rupture to leave:
- Ulcers round, painful, shallow (Figure 4.81).

Diagnosis

The clinical picture mimics primary herpetic stomatitis, but there is no gingivitis, and only moderate cervical lymphadenitis.

Management

Ulcers heal spontaneously in 7–10 days. Symptomatic treatment (Tables 10.1 and 10.2; see Herpes simplex, page 139).

Herpes simplex infections

Definition

Herpes simplex virus (HSV), infection is common and affects mainly the mouth (HSV type 1), or genitals or anus (HSV-2). All herpesvirus infections are characterized by latency, and can be reactivated during immunosuppression.

Incidence

Common

Age mainly affected

Children

Sex mainly affected

M=F

Aetiology

Herpes simplex virus, a DNA virus, contracted from infected saliva or other body fluids after an incubation period of approximately 4–7 days. Primary herpetic stomatitis (gingivostomatitis) is typically a childhood infection seen between the ages of 2–4 years (Figure 4.82), but cases are increasingly seen in older patients. Some of these are due to HSV-2 transmitted sexually. Some 50% of HSV infections are subclinical.

Clinical features

Primary herpetic stomatitis

Primary herpetic stomatitis presents with a single episode of:

* Oral vesicles which may be widespread (Figure 4.83), and break down to leave:

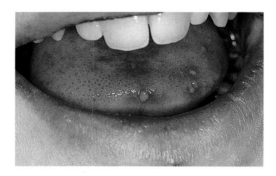

Figure 4.82
Herpes simplex infection: multiple ulcers in many sites

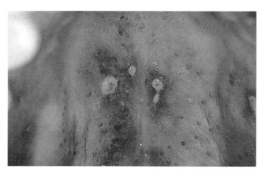

Figure 4.83
Herpes simplex infection: palatal vesicles

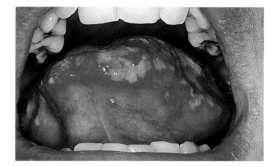

Figure 4.84
Herpes simplex infection: multiple ulcers

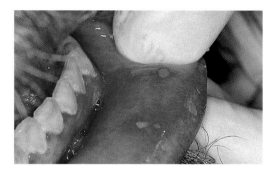

Figure 4.85
Herpes simplex infection

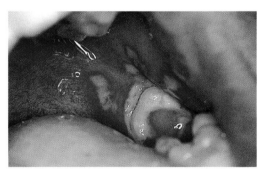

Figure 4.86
Herpes simplex infection: multiple painful ulcers on all mucosae

- Oral ulcers that are initially pinpoint but fuse to produce irregular painful ulcers (Figures 4.84–4.86);
- Gingival oedema, erythema and ulceration are prominent (Figures 4.87 and 4.88). Herpetic stomatitis probably explains many instances of 'teething';
- Tongue is often coated (Figure 4.89) and there is halitosis;
- Malaise and fever;
- Cervical lymph node enlargement.

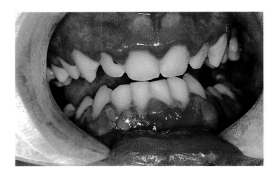

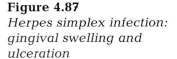

Figure 4.87
*Herpes simplex infection:
gingival swelling and
ulceration*

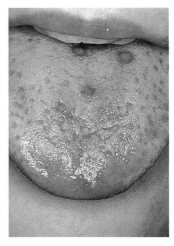

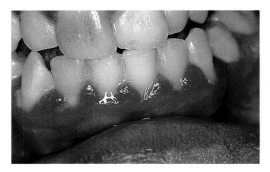

Figure 4.89
*Herpes simplex infection
producing ulcers and a
coated tongue*

Figure 4.88
Herpes simplex infection

Rare complications of primary HSV infection include encephalitis and mononeuropathies.

Recurrent herpetic infections

HSV-1 remains latent thereafter in the trigeminal ganglion but can be reactivated. Factors that can reactivate the virus include:

- Fever;
- Sunlight;
- Trauma;
- Immunosuppression.

There may be clinical recrudescence, recurrently, to produce herpes labialis or, occasionally, intraoral ulceration and virus is shed into saliva. Up to 15% of the normal, adult population have recurrent HSV-1 infections which present as:

- Lip lesions at the mucocutaneous junction; macules that rapidly turn papular, vesicular, then become pustular, scab and heal without scarring (Figures 4.90–4.92, 7.2, 7.24 and 7.25). Widespread

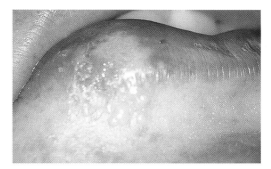

Figure 4.90
*Herpes simplex
infection: recurrent
herpes labialis at an
early stage*

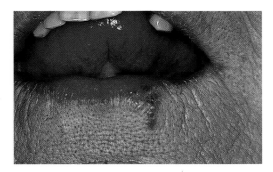

Figure 4.91
*Herpes simplex
infection: healing herpes
labialis*

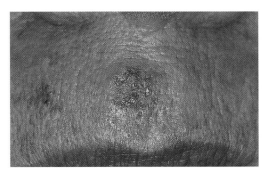

Figure 4.92
*Herpes simplex
infection: recurrence on
upper lip*

   recalcitrant lesions may appear in immunocompromised patients;
- Recurrent intraoral herpes in healthy patients tends to affect the hard palate or gingiva, as a small crop of ulcers usually over the greater palatine foramen, often following a palatal local anaesthetic injection, presumably because of the trauma. Lesions heal within 1–2 weeks (Figures 4.93 and 4.94);
- Recurrent intraoral herpes in immunocompromised patients may appear as chronic, often dendritic, ulcers frequently on the tongue (herpetic geometric glossitis). Clinical diagnosis tends to underestimate the frequency of these lesions (Figure 4.95).

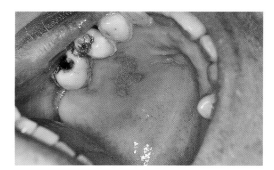

Figure 4.93
Herpes simplex infection: intraoral recurrence

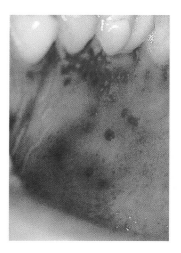

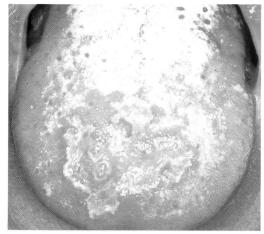

Figure 4.94
Recurrent herpes simplex infection

Figure 4.95
Herpes simplex infection: intraoral recurrence in immunocompromised patient

Diagnosis

Primary stomatitis

Diagnosis is largely clinical, although viral culture, immunodetection or electron microscopy are used occasionally. A rising titre of serum antibodies is confirmatory but only gives the diagnosis retrospectively.

Recurrent intraoral herpes

Diagnosis of recurrent intraoral herpes in healthy patients is largely clinical, although viral culture, immunodetection, PCR (polymerase chain reaction) or electron microscopy are used very occasionally. Assay of serum antibodies gives little help.

Diagnosis of recurrent intraoral herpes in immunocompromised patients is difficult, and viral culture, immunodetection, PCR or electron microscopy may be needed. Assay of serum antibodies gives little help.

Management

Primary stomatitis

- A soft diet and adequate fluid intake;
- Antipyretics/analgesics such as paracetamol elixir help relieve pain and fever;
- Local antiseptics (0.2% aqueous chlorhexidine mouthwashes) may aid resolution;
- Aciclovir orally or parenterally is useful in immunocompromised patients. Valaciclovir or famciclovir may be needed for aciclovir-resistant infections.

Recurrent intraoral herpes

Symptomatic treatment with a soft diet and adequate fluid intake, antipyretics/analgesics (paracetamol elixir), local antiseptics (0.2% aqueous chlorhexidine mouthwashes) usually suffices (Tables 10.1–10.11). Systemic aciclovir or other antivirals may be needed for immunocompromised patients.

Recurrent herpes labialis (see Chapter 7)

Histoplasmosis

Definition

A deep mycosis caused by *Histoplasma capsulatum*

Incidence

Uncommon, but histoplasmosis is the most frequently diagnosed systemic mycosis in the USA.

Age mainly affected

Adults

Sex mainly affected

M=F

Aetiology

Spores are found especially in bird and bat faeces, and soil particularly in north-eastern and central USA in Missouri, Kentucky, Tennessee, Illinois, Indiana and Ohio (mainly in the Ohio and Mississippi valleys), in Latin America, India, the Far East and in Australia.

Clinical features

- In endemic areas over 70% of adults appear to be infected, typically subclinically;
- Acute and chronic pulmonary and cutaneous histoplasmosis are the most common forms of clinical disease;
- In immunocompromised persons, there may be:
  - dissemination to the reticuloendothelial system, lungs, kidneys and gastrointestinal tract;
  - oral ulcerative or nodular lesions on the tongue, palate, buccal mucosa, gingiva or jaws.

Diagnosis

- Biopsy;
- Culture;
- Serotests.

The histoplasmin skin test is of little importance diagnostically.

Management

Amphotericin, ketoconazole, fluconazole or itraconazole (Table 10.8)

Human immunodeficiency virus (HIV) infection

Definition

Infection with human immunodeficiency viruses (HIV), which eventually results in immunodeficiency

Incidence

Increasing worldwide, especially in Asia. By 2001, probably 40 million persons were infected. Most infections worldwide are sexually transmitted, mainly by heterosexual sex and are seen in developing countries. HIV may also be transmitted in blood and blood products, by homosexual sex, and is increasingly common in intravenous drug users.

Age mainly affected

Young adults

Sex mainly affected

M>F in the developed world, but worldwide both sexes equally affected

Aetiology

Infection with human immunodeficiency retroviruses (RNA), damages T helper lymphocytes known as CD4 cells, and other CD4$^+$ cells

Clinical features

HIV may cause an initial glandular-fever-like illness but may be asymptomatic. The incubation period may extend over 5 or more years. HIV infection may be asymptomatic initially, even for months or years, but eventually infections with viruses, fungi and mycobacteria supervene, and patients may develop virally related neoplasms such as Kaposi's sarcoma, lymphoma and cervical or anal carcinoma, as well as autoimmune phenomena. As the CD4 cell count falls, the degree of immunoincompetence increases, and the patient develops opportunistic infections (from commensal organisms such as *Candida*), and may contract exogenous pathogens (such as TB) (Figure 4.96). The prognosis is almost invariably poor, with an extremely high mortality, albeit after a number of years in many cases. Oral features, none of which are absolutely specific for HIV infection, may include:

Candidiasis

Thrush (Figure 4.97) and erythematous (Figure 4.98) candidiasis, is an AIDS-defining disease seen in over 60% of AIDS patients, often as an early manifestation. It is the most common oral feature of HIV-related disease and may be a predictor of other opportunistic infections and of oesophageal thrush. Xerostomia and smoking may predispose to candidiasis. Infection may be controlled with antifungals.

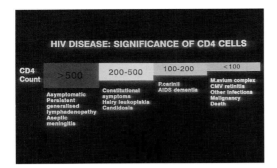

Figure 4.96
Human immunodeficiency virus infection: relationship of manifest disease with CD4 cell counts

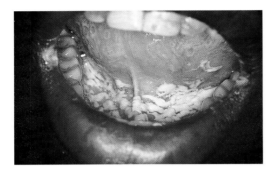

Figure 4.97
Human immunodeficiency virus infection resulting in oral thrush in an African patient

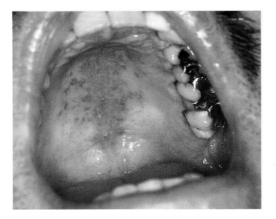

Figure 4.98
Human immunodeficiency virus infection producing erythematous candidiasis in a man who had sex with a man

Hairy leukoplakia

Hairy leukoplakia is a common, corrugated (or 'hairy') AIDS-defining white lesion usually seen on the lateral margins of the tongue (Figure 4.99). Hairy leukoplakia may be associated with Epstein–Barr virus (EBV) and may resolve with antivirals. Hairy leukoplakia is not known to be premalignant but it is a predictor of bad prognosis.

Kaposi's sarcoma

Kaposi's sarcoma presents as red, blue or purple macules, papules, nodules or ulcers and typically occurs at the hard/soft palate junction (Figure 4.100) or the anterior maxillary gingivae. Kaposi's sarcoma is seen mainly in sexually transmitted AIDS, may be associated with HHV-8 (human herpesvirus 8), and treated with chemotherapy.

Gingival and periodontal disease

Ulcerative gingivitis, and destructive periodontitis (Figure 4.101) can be features of HIV infection. Improved oral hygiene, debridement, chlorhexidine and sometimes metronidazole are needed.

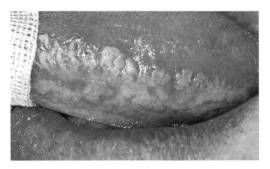

Figure 4.99
Human immunodeficiency virus infection: hairy leukoplakia – an AIDS-defining condition

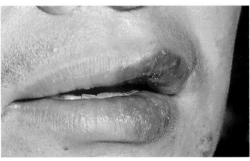

Figure 4.100
Human immunodeficiency virus infection: Kaposi's sarcoma is an AIDS-defining condition

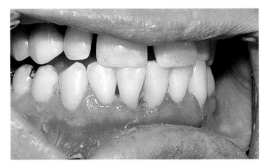

Figure 4.101
Human immunodeficiency virus infection: necrotising gingivitis

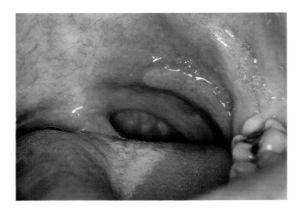

Figure 4.102
Human immunodeficiency virus infection: mouth ulceration

Ulcers

Aphthous-type ulcers, especially of the major type, may appear in HIV disease (Figure 4.102). Mouth ulcers are also occasionally caused by opportunistic pathogens such as herpesviruses, mycobacteria, histoplasma or cryptococcus. Antimicrobials are usually indicated.

Other orofacial lesions may include

- Cervical lymph node enlargement;
- Lymphomas (particularly non-Hodgkin's lymphomas);
- Cranial neuropathies;
- Parotitis, cystic salivary lesions and xerostomia;
- Human papillomavirus (HPV) infections and, in particular, genital warts (condyloma acuminata) in the mouth.

Oral lesions in HIV disease have been classified as follows:
Group I: lesions strongly associated with HIV infection:

- Candidiasis (erythematous, hyperplastic, thrush);
- Hairy leukoplakia (EBV);
- HIV-gingivitis;
- Necrotizing ulcerative gingivitis;
- HIV-periodontitis;
- Kaposi's sarcoma;
- Non-Hodgkin's lymphoma.

Group II: lesions less-commonly associated with HIV infection:

- Atypical ulceration (oropharyngeal);
- Idiopathic thrombocytopenic purpura;
- Salivary gland diseases (dry mouth, and unilateral or bilateral swelling of major salivary glands);

- Viral infections other than EBV (cytomegalovirus, herpes simplex virus, human papillomavirus (warty-like lesions—condyloma acuminatum, focal epithelial hyperplasia and verruca vulgaris), varicella-zoster virus: herpes zoster and varicella).

Group III: lesions possibly associated with HIV infection:

- A miscellany of diseases.

Diagnosis

Diagnosis can be straightforward such as when the patient has obvious lesions such as hairy leukoplakia, candidiasis and Kaposi's sarcoma, particularly if more than one lesion is present or if the patient is at especially high risk—such as an intravenous drug user or promiscuous homosexual. Nevertheless, serological confirmation is required but should be carried out only after appropriate counselling. In other cases, the diagnosis is far less clear-cut, particularly in a person apparently not at especial risk who has a single and common lesion such as an apthous-type of ulcer.

Management

Considerable compassion is called for. Specialist care will be required at some stage in virtually all patients. Treatment with antiretroviral agents is increasingly effective at controlling the decline in CD4 cells, and clinical manifestations. Zidovudine (ZDI, sometimes termed AZT) was the first and only available anti-HIV therapy for several years, but other nucleoside inhibitors of the HIV enzyme reverse transcriptase (NRTIs) such as dideoxyinosine (didanosine, ddl), dideoxycytidine (zalcitabine, ddC), lamivudine (3TC) and stavudine (d4T) have been developed in the past decade, though all are liable to fairly severe adverse reactions and resistance. The last few years have seen considerable progress in anti-HIV therapy, with the introduction of the HIV non-nucleoside reverse transcriptase inhibitors (efavirenz, delaviradine and nevaripine) (NNRTIs) and later the HIV protease inhibitors (PIs) such as saquinavir, indinavir, ritonavir and nelfinavir, which proved to be a major advance. There has latterly been extraordinary progress in developing combination therapies against HIV, such as highly active antiretroviral therapies (HAART). These have reduced the incidence of infections and have extended life substantially but now that there are at least 15 antiretroviral agents available, the therapy of HIV has become extremely complex. One of the main problems with all antiretroviral agents has been the associated adverse effects, some of which affect the orofacial region, causing especially:

- Taste disturbances;
- Paraesthesia;

- Dry mouth;
- Ulceration.

Infections and tumours should be treated as described elsewhere in this book.

Infectious mononucleosis (Paul–Bunnell positive glandular fever)

Definition

Infectious mononucleosis (IM) is characterized by sore throat, lymphadenopathy and malaise with a positive Paul–Bunnell test result.

Incidence

Uncommon except in adolescents

Age mainly affected

Adolescents and young adults

Sex mainly affected

M=F

Aetiology

Epstein–Barr virus (EBV) transmitted in saliva ('kissing disease')

Clinical features

The incubation of 30–50 days is followed by:

- Fever;
- Malaise;
- Generalized tender lymphadenopathy;

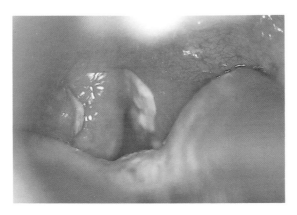

Figure 4.103
Infectious mononucleosis: substantial faucial oedema and exudates

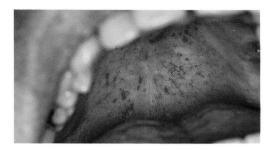

Figure 4.104
*Infectious mononucleosis:
palatal petechiae*

- Sore throat and tonsillar exudate (Figure 4.103). There is severe dysphagia and faucial oedema can, rarely, obstruct the airway.

Oral features in IM may include:

- Palatal petechiae, especially at the junction of the hard and soft palate, are almost pathognomonic but can be seen in other viral infections such as HIV and rubella, and in noninfective causes of thrombocytopathy (Figure 4.104);
- Mouth ulcers.

EBV may also cause persistent malaise, and has associations with lymphomas and other neoplasms, and hairy leukoplakia.

Diagnosis

Several other conditions which may present similarly (glandular-fever-like syndromes) include HIV infection, cytomegalovirus infection, herpesvirus-6 infection, *Toxoplasma gondii* infection and diphtheria (Table 4.11).

Investigations required include a blood picture, the Paul–Bunnell test for heterophil antibodies (positive in IM) and sometimes other tests.

Table 4.11   Glandular fever syndromes

	Causal agents				
	Epstein–Barr virus (EBV)	*Cytomegalo-virus (CMV)*	*Human immune deficiency viruses (HIV)*	*Toxo-plasma gondii*	*Human herpesvirus-6*
Blood investigations to confirm infection	Paul–Bunnell test, EBV serum antibodies	CMV serum antibodies	HIV serum antibody titres Lymphopenia T4 (CD4) cell numbers	Sabin–Feldman dye test Specific IgM serum antibodies	HHV-6 serum antibodies

Management

Symptomatic treatment for oral lesions (see Herpes simplex, page 139) is usually all that can be offered, though metronidazole may improve the sore throat. Many patients require bed rest because of the profound fatigue.

Keratoses

Frictional keratosis

Definition

White lesion caused by repeated trauma

Incidence

Common

Age mainly affected

Middle-aged and elderly

Sex mainly affected

M>F

Aetiology

Frictional keratosis is caused by prolonged mild abrasion by such irritants as a sharp tooth, denture, or cheek biting. An occlusal line (linea alba) is often seen in the buccal mucosae. Cheek biting (morsicatio buccarum) is most prevalent in anxious females, especially those with other psychologically related disorders. Rarely self-mutilation is seen in psychiatric disorders, learning disability or some rare syndromes (Figure 1.26).

Clinical features

In the early stages, the patch is pale and translucent, later becoming dense and white, sometimes with a rough surface. A linea alba may

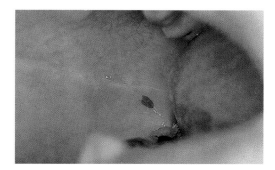

Figure 4.105
Frictional keratosis at the occlusal line (linear alba)

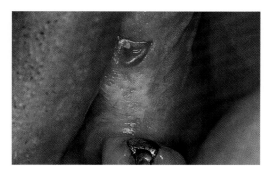

Figure 4.106
Frictional keratosis on the alveolar ridge

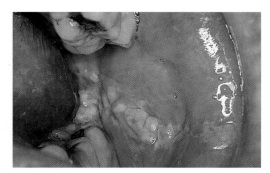

Figure 4.107
Cheek biting: keratosis only around the occlusal line

be seen in isolation (Figure 4.105) or sometimes with crenation of the lateral margins of the tongue, from pressure. The occlusal line is typically thin, white and there are occasional petechiae. Keratoses are not uncommonly seen on edentulous ridges, especially in the partially dentate, and then presumably caused by the friction from mastication (Figure 4.106). Habitual cheek biting causes red and white lesions with a rough surface, invariably restricted to the lower labial and/or buccal mucosa near the occlusal line (Figures 4.59 and 4.107).

Diagnosis

The diagnosis is clinical and, apart from removing irritants and ceasing habits, no active treatment is required.

Management

Frictional keratosis is completely benign and does not require treatment. There is no evidence that continued minor trauma alone has any carcinogenic potential; however, if the patient is causing the lesion from some habit, that should be stopped.

Sublingual keratosis (see Chapter 9)

Tobacco-related keratoses (Smoker's keratosis (see Chapter 8), Snuff dippers' keratosis and other smokeless tobacco lesions)

Definition

White hyperkeratotic lesions caused by tobacco-chewing or snuff-dipping

Incidence

Uncommon

Age mainly affected

Adults

Sex mainly affected

M=F

Aetiology

Tobacco-chewing or snuff-dipping (holding flavoured tobacco powder in the oral sulcus or vestibule) causes white oedematous and hyperkeratotic wrinkled white plaque lesions in up to 20% of users. Oral snuff appears to cause more severe clinical changes than does

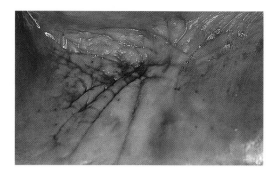

Figure 4.108
*Snuff-induced keratosis
in the vestibule*

tobacco-chewing, but dysplasia is more likely in tobacco chewers. Snuff-dipping is associated predominantly with verrucous keratoses which can progress to verrucous carcinoma, but only after several decades of use.

Clinical features

There is typically a white lesion in the buccal sulcus, and a high proportion of the tumours are seen in the buccal mucosa/vestibule (Figure 4.108). The lesions appear adjacent to where the snuff is placed and there may be some gingival recession.

Diagnosis

The diagnosis is usually obvious from the habit.

Management

Snuff dippers' lesions usually resolve on stopping the habit, even after years of use. Biopsy may be indicated.

Chronic hyperplastic candidiasis (candidal leukoplakia)

Definition

This term applies to lesions consisting of white flecks, plaques or fine nodules often on an atrophic erythematous base (speckled leukoplakia), which will not wipe off with a gauze. It is regarded as a combination of, or transition between, leukoplakia and erythro-plasia (see below) associated with candidal infection.

Incidence

Uncommon

Age mainly affected

Middle-aged and elderly

Sex mainly affected

M=F

Aetiology

Candida albicans can produce nitrosamines and can induce epithelial proliferation. Smoking appears to predispose to this lesion.

Clinical features

Chronic oral candidiasis produces a tough adherent white plaque, distinguishable only by biopsy from other leukoplakia-like condi-tions. The usual sites are the dorsum of the tongue and the postcom-missural buccal mucosa (Figures 4.48 and 4.109). The plaque is vari-able in thickness and often rough or irregular in texture, or nodular with an erythematous background (speckled leukoplakia). Candidal leukoplakias may be potentially malignant.

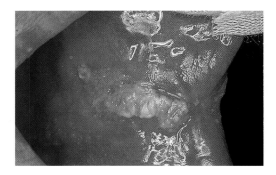

Figure 4.109
Candidal leukoplakia in a typical site

Diagnosis

Unlike acute candidiasis (thrush), the plaque cannot be wiped off, but fragments can be detached by firm scraping. Gram-staining then shows candidal hyphae embedded in clumps of detached epithelial cells. However, biopsy is indicated in view of the possibility of dysplasia.

Management

- The patient should stop smoking;
- Antifungal treatment is indicated;
- If the lesion does not resolve it is probably better to remove it by excision, laser or cryosurgery.

Syphilitic leukoplakia (see page 224)

Carcinoma

Oral squamous cell carcinoma may present as an innocuous-looking white patch.

Koilocytic dysplasia

This is a pathological description of a papillomavirus-associated lesion that presents as a flat or elevated white lesion seen in the lingual, buccal or labial mucosa, sometimes in HIV-infected individuals. HPV 6/11, 16/18 or 31/33/51 are implicated; the prognosis is uncertain but there are some features of dysplasia.

Langerhans' cell histiocytoses

Definition

Neoplasms arising from Langerhans' cells (dendritic intraepithelial macrophage-like cells)

Incidence

Rare

Age mainly affected

From childhood

Sex mainly affected

M=F

Aetiology

Unknown; malignant neoplasm affecting CD1a-positive cells

Clinical features

Langerhan's cell histiocytoses are a group of disorders, formerly termed histiocytosis X, including:

- Solitary eosinophilic granuloma (chronic localized Langerhans' cell histiocytosis): usually a localized benign form seen mainly in young male adults characterized by:
  - A solitary ulcer and osteolytic lesion only;
  - Mainly seen in posterior mandible;
  - Gross periodontal destruction;
  - The affected teeth may loosen.

- Multifocal or chronic disseminated eosinophilic granuloma: Hand–Schuller–Christian disease is a more malignant form in children and young adults characterized by:
  - Ulcers and osteolytic lesions;
  - Loosening of teeth (floating teeth);
  - Diabetes insipidus;
  - Proptosis.

- Letterer–Siwe disease or acute disseminated Langerhan's cell histiocytosis: an acute disseminated and usually lethal form in infants characterized by:
  - Failure to thrive;
  - Fever;
  - Hepatosplenomegaly;
  - Ulcers and osteolytic lesions that may cause pain;
  - Loosening of teeth.

Diagnosis

Clinical features, radiography and histology

Management

- Curettage suffices for chronic localized forms;
- Chemo- and/or radiotherapy are required for disseminated forms.

Leukaemia

Definition

Malignant proliferation of leukocytes

Incidence

Uncommon

Age mainly affected

50–60% of leukaemias are acute, affecting mainly children or young adults. Chronic myeloid leukaemia is seen mainly in middle-aged adults; chronic lymphocytic leukaemia is seen mainly in the elderly.

Sex mainly affected

M=F

Aetiology

Ionizing radiation, immunosuppression, chemicals, chromosomal disorders, retroviruses (rarely)

Clinical features

- Oral purpura (Figure 4.110);
- Spontaneous gingival haemorrhage (and prolonged post-extraction bleeding);
- Mouth ulcers; associated with cytotoxic therapy, with viral, bacterial or fungal infection or nonspecific (Figure 4.111);

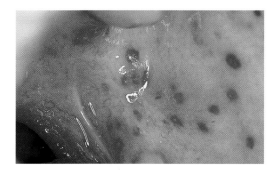

Figure 4.110
Leukaemia: oral purpura

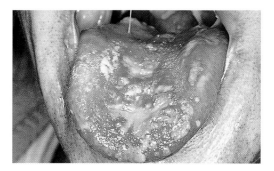

Figure 4.111
Leukaemia: recurrent oral herpes simplex virus ulceration

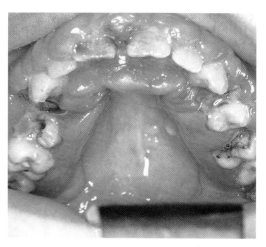

Figure 4.112
Leukaemia: gingival swelling

- Leukaemic deposits occasionally cause swelling; gingival swelling is a feature especially of myelomonocytic leukaemia (Figure 4.112);
- Microbial infections, mainly fungal and viral are common in the mouth and can be a significant problem. Candidiasis is extremely

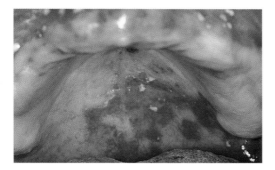

Figure 4.113
Leukaemia: candidiasis

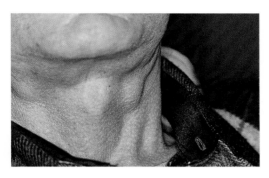

Figure 4.114
*Leukaemia: cervical and
other lymph nodes are
enlarged*

common (Figure 4.113). Recurrent intraoral herpes simplex (Figure 4.111) or herpes labialis is also common. Mucoromycosis and aspergillosis may be seen;
- Simple odontogenic infections can spread widely and be difficult to control;
- Non-odontogenic oral infections can involve a range of bacteria including *Staphylococcus aureus*, *Pseudomonas aeruginosa*, *Klebsiella pneumoniae*, *Staphylococcus epidermidis*, *Escherichia coli* and enterococci;
- Cervical and generalized lymph node enlargement (Figure 4.114).

Diagnosis

Blood picture and marrow biopsy

Management

- Cytotoxic chemotherapy, highly successful in childhood leukaemias;
- Oral health care (Tables 10.1 and 10.2);
- Management of oral infections.

Leukoedema

Definition

A benign congenital whitish filmy appearance of the mucosa

Incidence

Common: seen in 85% Blacks, 45% Caucasians

Age mainly affected

Any

Sex mainly affected

M=F

Aetiology

Congenital increase in intracellular glycogen in stratum spinosum

Clinical features

A whitish filmy appearance particularly seen in the buccal mucosae bilaterally; the white appearance disappears if the mucosa is stretched (Figure 4.115).

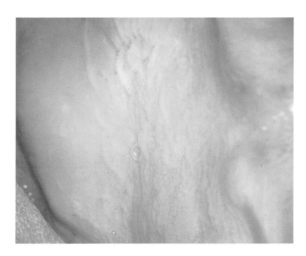

Figure 4.115
Leukoedema (plus friction and ulceration)

Diagnosis

Diagnosis is clinical.

Management

Reassurance only is required.

Leukopenia

Definition

Reduction in leukocyte count

Incidence

Rare

Age mainly affected

Adults

Sex mainly affected

M=F

Aetiology

Viral infections, drugs, irradiation, idiopathic

Clinical features

Predisposition to:

- Infections: mucosal, periodontal, systemic or postoperative;
- Ulcers: persistent ulcers lacking inflammatory halo.

Diagnosis

- Full blood picture;
- Bone marrow biopsy.

Management

- Improve oral hygiene;
- Antimicrobials as necessary.

Leukoplakia

Idiopathic (including dysplastic) leukoplakia

Definition

Leukoplakias are white patches that cannot be wiped off the mucosa and that have no identifiable aetiology.

Incidence

Relatively common; up to 5% of adults older than 40 years

Age mainly affected

M=F

Aetiology

No specific aetiological factor can be identified for the majority of persistent oral white plaques, which are thus termed *idiopathic* leukoplakias, but most other affected patients smoke tobacco and/or drink alcohol.

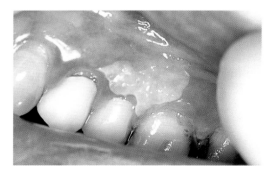

Figure 4.116
Leukoplakia;
homogeneous benign flat
white plaque

Clinical features

- Most leukoplakias are benign smooth white plaques (homogeneous leukoplakias) (Figures 4.116 and 4.117);
- Most are seen on the lip, buccal mucosae or gingivae;
- Some are white and warty (verrucous leukoplakia) (Figure 4.118);
- Some are mixed white and red lesions (speckled leukoplakias) (Figure 4.119) with a high malignant potential;
- Some are potentially malignant. Dysplasia appears currently to be the best predictor of malignant potential. Up to 10% of leukoplakias

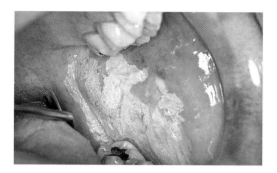

Figure 4.117
Leukoplakia;
homogeneous (usually
benign)

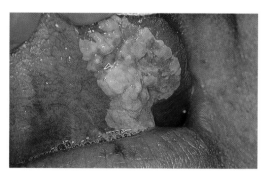

Figure 4.118
Leukoplakia; nodular
(sometimes potentially
malignant)

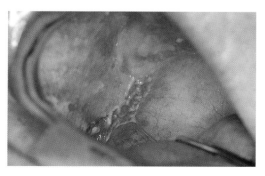

Figure 4.119
Leukoplakia; speckled
(erythroleukoplakia:
highest malignant
potential of all
leukoplakias)

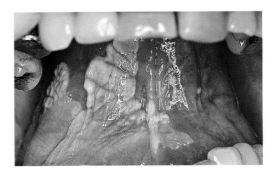

Figure 4.120
*Leukoplakia; floor of
mouth (sublingual)*

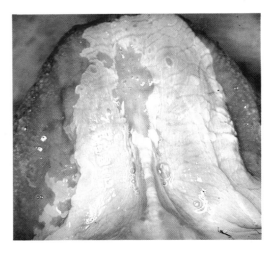

Figure 4.121
*Leukoplakia; floor of
mouth (sublingual)*

are dysplastic at the first visit. Dysplastic lesions do not have any specific clinical appearance, although where erythroplasia is present, dysplasia, carcinoma in situ or frank carcinomas may be seen. Site is relevant; leukoplakias in the floor of mouth/ventrum of tongue and lip are sinister (Figures 4.120, 4.121 and 9.32–9.34).

Size appears irrelevant. Small and innocent-looking white patches are as likely to show epithelial dysplasia as are large and irregular ones. Even small dysplastic lesions can be followed by multiple carcinomas and a fatal outcome.

The most extensive follow-up studies suggest that idiopathic leukoplakia has the highest risk of developing cancer. Up to 10% of those with moderate and 30% of those with severe dysplasia develop carcinoma in a 10 year period. Malignant change appears to be more frequent among nonsmokers. The prognosis thus appears worse for:

- Lesions in high-risk sites such as floor of mouth;

- Nonsmokers;
- Females;
- Where there is dysplasia;
- Where there are multiple recurrent verrucous lesions (proliferative verrucous leukoplakia).

Diagnosis

- Clinical;
- Biopsy. Selecting the most appropriate area to biopsy is not easy; guidance can be obtained by selecting any *red* area, or using a vital stain such as toluidine blue to highlight areas.

Management

- The management of leukoplakias is far from satisfactory and there are no large trials that offer guidance as to the most reliable treatment;
- Certainly any causal factor should be corrected where possible. Tobacco and alcohol habits should be stopped;
- Any degree of dysplasia in a lesion at a high-risk site must be taken very seriously;
- Experts remove dysplastic lesions, where possible, surgically with scalpel, laser or cryoprobe;
- Retinoids are currently being investigated as a possible treatment modality; they appear very effective, but their beneficial effect appears to last only during the treatment and their drawbacks are severe adverse effects on liver function and teratogenicity;
- Occasionally patients are treated by photodynamic therapy or topical cytotoxic agents;
- The patient should be monitored regularly (at 3–6 months intervals).

Lichen planus

Definition

Lichen planus (LP) is a common mucocutaneous disorder characterized in some by oral white lesions and sometimes genital lesions and/or an itchy rash mainly on the wrists.

Incidence

Common

Age mainly affected

Middle-aged and elderly

Sex mainly affected

F>M

Aetiology

Unclear, though there is clear evidence of a T lymphocyte attack on the stratified squamous epithelia (Figure 4.122). A minority of cases are related to the following:

- Drugs. Lichen-planus-like (lichenoid) lesions may be induced by antihypertensives, antidiabetics, gold salts, nonsteroidal anti-inflammatory agents, antimalarials and other drugs. Suggested associations of oral LP with systemic disease such as diabetes mellitus and hypertension (Grinspan syndrome) are most probably explained by drug-induced lichenoid lesions;
- Reactions to amalgam or gold or occasionally other materials;
- Graft-versus-host disease;
- HIV infection;
- Hepatitis C virus infection.

There is a much lower prevalence of liver disease in oral lichen planus in the UK than has appeared in some reports from southern Europe and Japan.

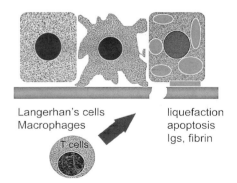

Langerhan's cells
Macrophages

T cells

liquefaction
apoptosis
Igs, fibrin

Figure 4.122
Lichen planus: a T lymphocyte-mediated lesion with keratinocyte apoptosis, liquefaction degeneration of the epithelial basement membrane and non-specific immune deposits of fibrin and immunoglobulins (Igs) in keratinocytes (colloid or Russell bodies)

Clinical features

The oral lesions of lichen planus are typically bilateral, posterior, in the buccal (cheek) mucosa, sometimes the tongue or gingivae, and rarely on the palate.

Lesions may be asymptomatic or may cause soreness, especially if atrophic or erosive. Some may be associated with hyperpigmentation, especially in non-caucasians. Presentations include:

- A network of raised white lines or striae (reticular pattern) (Figure 4.123);
- White papules (Figure 4.124);
- White plaques, simulating leukoplakia (Figure 4.125);

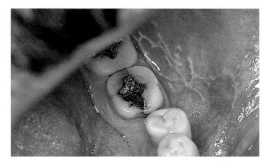

Figure 4.123
Lichen planus: reticular lesions in the most common site

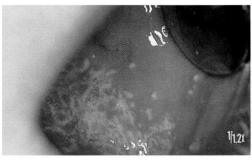

Figure 4.124
Lichen planus: papular lesions may mimic candidiasis

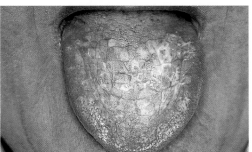

Figure 4.125
Lichen planus: reticular and plaque-like lesions may be mistaken for leukoplakia

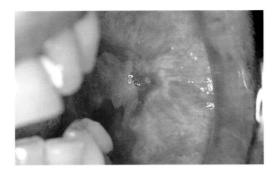

Figure 4.126
Lichen planus: erosive type can cause considerable discomfort

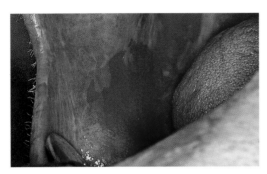

Figure 4.127
Lichen planus: atrophic form may closely resemble erythroplasia

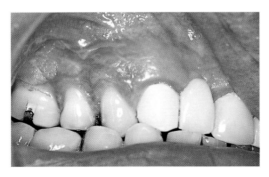

Figure 4.128
Lichen planus: affecting gingiva

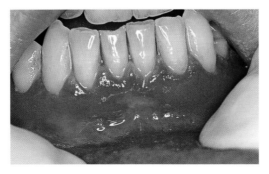

Figure 4.129
Lichen planus: desquamative gingivitis

- Erosions are less common, persistent, irregular and painful with a yellowish slough (Figure 4.126) plus white lesions;
- Red atrophic areas (Figure 4.127);
- Lichen planus may cause atrophic lesions plus white lesions (Figure 4.128) and is one of the most common cause of desquamative gingivitis (Figure 4.129);

LP may also affect the following:

- Skin: with itchy (pruritic), purple, polygonal, papules (small raised rash) especially on the flexor surface of the wrists (Figures 4.130 and 4.131). Trauma may induce lesions (Koebner phenomenon);
- Genitals: with white or erosive lesions;
- Nails: ridging;
- Hair: loss.

Lichenoid lesions resemble LP but may:

- Often be unilateral (Figure 4.132);
- Affect particularly the palate and tongue;
- Be associated with erosions;
- Resolve on discontinuation of the offending drug or removal of the causal material.

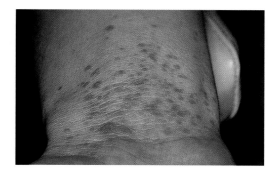

Figure 4.130
Lichen planus in a typical site on the flexor surfaces of the forearms

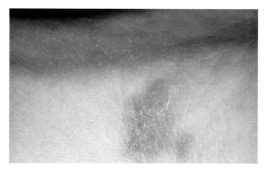

Figure 4.131
Lichen planus showing white Wickham's striae

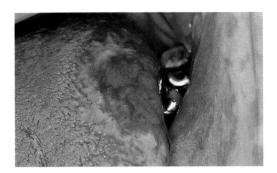

Figure 4.132
*Lichenoid lesions related
to dental restorations*

Diagnosis

The history and clinical appearance are usually highly indicative of the
diagnosis but lesional biopsy is often indicated, particularly to exclude:

- Lupus erythematosus;
- Leukoplakia (keratosis);
- Malignancy.

Specialist referral may be indicated if for example:

- The diagnosis is uncertain;
- Oral lesions are recalcitrant;
- There is concern about malignancy;
- There are extraoral lesions.

Histological features include:

- A dense subepithelial cellular infiltrate including many T lym-
  phocytes;
- Hyperkeratosis;
- Colloid bodies in the epithelium;
- Basal cell liquefaction degeneration;
- Immunostaining for fibrin at the basement membrane zone.

Lichenoid lesions are more likely than LP to be associated with:

- A mixed cellular infiltrate including many plasma cells and
  eosinophils;
- A deeper and less sharply defined infiltrate;
- A perivascular infiltrate;
- Parakeratosis;
- Colloid bodies in the epithelium;
- Basal cell autoantibodies;
- Considerable basal cell liquefaction degeneration.

Oral LP is often persistent but is usually benign. Clinically, atrophic LP closely resembles erythroplasia, a premalignant condition, and there is about a 1–3% chance of malignant transformation over 5 years, predominantly in those with long-standing LP.

Management

- Predisposing factors (such as amalgam or gold restorations), should be excluded. If amalgams might be implicated, it may be worthwhile considering a trial, changing amalgams adjacent to lesions for an alternative material;
- If drugs are implicated, the physician should be consulted about possible changes in therapy;
- Oral hygiene should be improved (Tables 10.1 and 10.2);
- Symptomatic oral LP may respond to topical corticosteroids but typically the more potent agents such as beclomethasone dipropionate, fluticasone or budesonide are required (Chapter 10). Antifungals may also be helpful (Tables 10.5 and 10.8);
- Recalcitrant mucosal lesions can be managed with intralesional corticosteroids or topical cyclosporin or tacrolimus;
- Recalcitrant gingival lesions can be managed with topical corticosteroid creams held in place overnight by a soft plastic splint;
- Systemic immunosuppressive agents including corticosteroids, azathioprine, cyclosporin or dapsone, or, rarely, vitamin A derivatives such as isotretinoin may be needed for widespread or severe LP (Table 10.7);
- Patients should stop smoking;
- Regular follow-up is indicated, especially in those with a higher risk of malignancy, long-standing erosive LP.

Lichenoid lesions

See page 173

Linear IgA disease

Definition

Linear IgA disease is a disorder very similar to dermatitis herpetiformis, but the lesional IgA deposits are linear at the epithelial basement membrane zone and with no C3, and there is no gluten-sensitive enteropathy.

Incidence

Rare

Age mainly affected

Adults, 5th or 6th decades; in children the same disease is termed chronic bullous disorder of childhood.

Sex mainly affected

M>F

Aetiology

Autoimmune or occasionally drug-induced (eg vancomycin)

Clinical features, Diagnosis and Management

See dermatitis herpetiformis (page 121)

Lipoma

This rare benign neoplasm presents as a slow-growing, spherical, smooth and soft semifluctuant lump with a characteristic yellowish colour caused by the fat that makes up the bulk of the lesion.

Lupus erythematosus

Definition

Lupus erythematosus is an autoimmune disease disorder with antibodies against nuclear components.

Incidence

Uncommon

Age mainly affected

Adults

Sex mainly affected

F>M

Aetiology

Lupus is an autoimmune multisystem disorder with antibodies against nuclear components. Precipitants may be drugs such as chlorpromazine, isonicofinic acid hydrazide, methyldopa, hydralazine or procainamide, and possibly environmental, hormonal and viral factors.

Clinical features

Both discoid (DLE) and systemic (SLE) lupus erythematosus can affect the mouth, and oral lesions can precede other manifestations in a minority of patients.

Discoid lupus erythematosus (DLE)

Oral manifestations of DLE are uncommon, and may mimic lichen planus with the following:

- Well-demarcated erythematous areas with a border of fine white striae, intermingled with prominent capillaries. The centre of the lesion may ulcerate, especially in those with DLE who will progress to SLE. Ulcers are more prevalent in those with active lupus;
- Lesions usually seen bilaterally on the labial, buccal or alveolar mucosae and the vermillion border (Figure 4.133);
- Labial lesions of DLE have a small malignant potential.

Systemic lupus erythematosus (SLE)

SLE is a multisystem disorder with lesions that may in particular involve:

- Skin; the characteristic rash is a 'butterfly rash' over the nose;
- Kidneys;
- CNS.

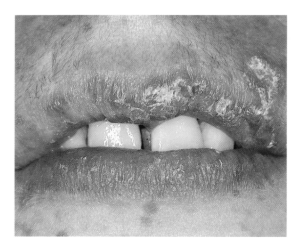

Figure 4.133
Discoid lupus erythematosus

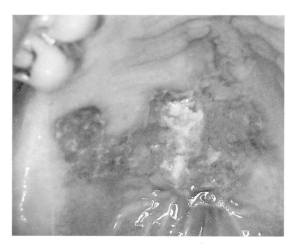

Figure 4.134
Systemic lupus erythematosus

Oral manifestations in SLE include:

- Painful erythematous patches;
- Nonspecific ulceration;
- Occasional keratotic patches particularly on the hard palate (Figure 4.134);
- Sjögren's syndrome.

Diagnosis

Differentiation of LE from LP in particular can be difficult or impossible.

- Serum autoantibodies, especially crithidial (double-stranded DNA) antinuclear antibodies, are present in SLE, not DLE or LP;
- Biopsy: histology shows significant atrophy, a deep and patchy lymphocytic infiltrate with flame-shaped rete processes and thickened basement membrane zone. The lupus band test shows immunoglobulin deposits at the basement membrane zone in epithelium. Granular deposits, mainly of IgM, are found at the basement membrane zone in most lesional and some 50% of clinically normal oral mucosa in SLE. Oral lesions of SLE with IgG, C3 or IgA deposits on immunostaining are more likely than those with IgM alone to predict cutaneous and renal involvement.

Management

- Topical corticosteroids can be effective in oral DLE but betamethasone cream rather than triamcinolone should be used (Table 10.5). Intralesional steroids may be required (Table 10.6);
- Isolated lesions can sometimes be excised or treated with cryoprobe;
- Recalcitrant lesions may respond to dapsone, antimalarials or systemic corticosteroids (Table 10.7);
- Oral lesions of SLE usually respond to conventional systemic treatment of SLE.

Lymphangioma

Definition

Hamartoma or benign neoplasm of lymphatic channels

Incidence

Rare

Age mainly affected

Seen from an early age

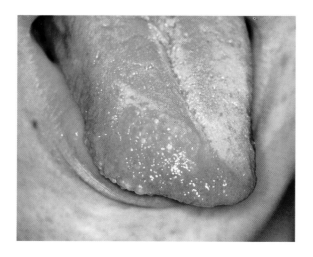

Figure 4.135
Lymphangioma

Sex mainly affected

M=F

Aetiology

Congenital

Clinical features

Lymphangiomas are seen mainly in the head and neck, especially in the tongue or lip (Figure 4.135). Most appear by the age of 2 years. Although typically a colourless sometimes finely nodular soft mass, bleeding into the lymphatic spaces causes sudden purplish discolouration. If in tongue and extensive, lymphangioma is a rare cause of macroglossia. If in lip, it is a rare cause of macrocheilia.

Diagnosis

Differentiate from haemangiomas mainly

Management

Excise for microscopy. Sclerosing agents tend not to produce resolution.

Lymphoma

Definition

Malignant neoplasm arising from lymphocytes

Incidence

Oral lymphomas are rare but, with the increase in HIV disease and other immunocompromised persons, are becoming more common.

Age mainly affected

Lymphomas are seen mainly in young adults. However, African Burkitt's lymphoma typically affects children before the age of 12–13 years.

Sex mainly affected

M>F

Aetiology

Lymphomas affecting the oral cavity are mainly B cell lymphomas. In HIV infection (mostly non-Hodgkin's lymphomas) and African Burkitt's lymphoma they are often associated with Epstein–Barr virus. T cell lymphomas are occasionally associated with HTLV-1.

Clinical features

Hodgkin's lymphoma

Hodgkin's disease affects males predominantly and has a bimodal distribution, being seen in late adolescence and in old age. It presents with:

- Enlarged rubbery lymph nodes, often in the neck;
- Fever, pruritus, weight loss and night sweats;
- In advanced disease also with hepatosplenomegaly.

Oral lesions are rare.

Non-Hodgkin's lymphoma

Non-Hodgkin's lymphomas (NHL) is predisposed by:

- HIV disease;
- Immunosuppression;
- Autoimmune disease.

NHL presents similarly to Hodgkin's disease but some may be extra-nodal and then may present with lumps or ulcers intraorally, especially in the fauces or maxillary gingivae, or with bony deposits, resulting in pain, anaesthesia, swelling, loosening of teeth or pathological fracture (Figures 4.136–4.138).

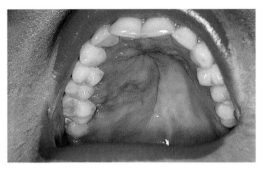

Figure 4.136
Lymphoma in a typical site

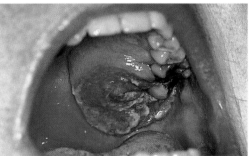

Figure 4.137
Lymphoma: most oral lymphomas are NHL

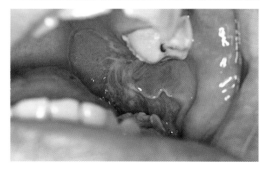

Figure 4.138
Lymphoma

Burkitt's lymphoma (BL)

The jaws are common sites of presentation of African BL. Massive swelling, which ulcerates in the mouth, pain, paraesthesia or increasing tooth mobility may result. Discrete radiolucencies especially in the lower third molar region, destruction of lamina dura and widening of the periodontal space or teeth which may appear to be 'floating in air', may be seen on radiography.

Polymorphic immunoblastic B lymphoproliferative disease

This presents as diffuse lumps or nodules, especially in the fauces or gingiva in HIV disease.

Diagnosis

Biopsy is required to establish the diagnosis.

Management

Chemotherapy and radiotherapy. HL now has a 50–90% 5-year survival; NHL has <50% 5-year survival.

Malignant ulcers

Most malignant oral ulcers are squamous cell carcinomas. Other primary tumours can be antral (rarely), or of salivary glands, or others, e.g. lymphomas, Kaposi's sarcoma or metastases. The incidence of carcinoma, lymphomas and Kaposi's sarcoma is rising, the latter two virus-related tumours because of the increasing incidence of AIDS.

Melanoacanthoma

Definition

Large brown macule

Incidence

Rare; seen mainly in Blacks

Age mainly affected

Adult, 3rd decade

Sex mainly affected

F>M

Aetiology

Reactive; often follows trauma

Clinical features

Usually:

- A dark brown macule;
- Asymptomatic;
- 1–3 cm diameter;
- Rough surface and sharply demarcated outline;
- Seen especially in buccal mucosa (Figure 4.139);
- Solitary and unilateral;
- Appears rapidly;
- Unchanging in character.

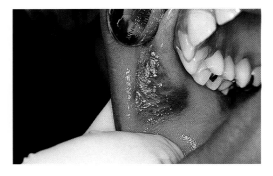

Figure 4.139
Melanoacanthoma

Diagnosis

May clinically resemble early melanoma, especially if it develops rapidly and therefore it should be biopsied for histopathological examination.

Management

Excise for diagnostic reasons.

Melanoma

Definition

Malignant neoplasm of melanocytes

Incidence

Rare; Japan and Uganda are areas of high risk.

Age mainly affected

Middle-aged and elderly

Sex mainly affected

M=F

Aetiology

Sunlight exposure is causal in skin melanomas, which have increased in almost epidemic fashion over the past decades, especially in fair-skinned peoples.

Clinical features

- Usually initially a solitary small asymptomatic brown or black macule;
- Typically seen on the hard palate or maxillary gingivae;
- Grows rapidly, initially spreading radially and superficially;
- Later becomes increasingly pigmented, nodular, deeply invasive and with satellite lesions (Figure 4.140).

Occasionally melanomas are nodular *ab initio* with deep spread, or are multiple or large. Up to 10% are nonpigmented.

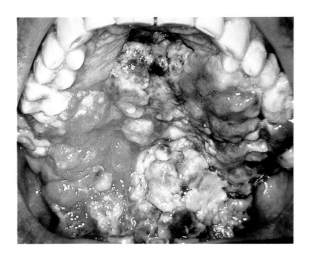

Figure 4.140
Malignant melanoma: seen mainly in the palate or maxillary alveolus

Diagnosis

The lesion should be excised for histopathological examination. Histopathologically, the mucosal epithelium is abnormal with large atypical melanocytes and excessive melanin. The lesion stains positively with S100, vimentin and HMB45 stains.

Management

- Melanomas which are less than about 0.75 mm thick are superficial and rarely metastasize, and can be excised in their entirety with a good prognosis;
- Others have a poor prognosis but can be excised; some centres use chemo- and immunotherapy.

Melanotic macule

Definition

Small brown macule; on the skin this would be called a freckle, lentigo or ephelis.

Incidence

Common

Age mainly affected

Adult

Sex mainly affected

F>M

Aetiology

Physiological or reactive

Clinical features

Usually:

- A very small brown macule;
- Asymptomatic;
- Seen especially on anterior gingivae (Figure 4.141), or lips;
- Solitary on the lip; may be multiple buccally (Figure 4.142);
- Unchanging in character.

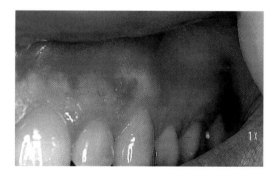

Figure 4.141
Melanotic macule

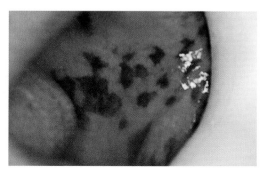

Figure 4.142
Melanotic macules: rarely, these can be multiple

Occasionally these grow rapidly or are multiple or large (melano-acanthoma).

Diagnosis

May clinically resemble early melanoma, especially if it develops rapidly, and therefore it should be excised for histopathological examination. Histopathologically, the mucosal epithelium is normal apart from increased pigmentation of the basal layer, accentuated at the tips of rete ridges. There is negative staining for HMB-45 (naevi are positive).

Management

Excise for diagnostic reasons.

Melanotic neuroectodermal tumour

Definition

Small brown nodule on anterior maxillary ridge in infant

Incidence

Rare

Age mainly affected

Infant

Sex mainly affected

M=F

Aetiology

Idiopathic

Clinical features

- A solitary nodule;
- May or may not be pigmented;
- Seen on anterior maxillary ridge;
- Grows rapidly;
- May destroy bone and displace teeth;
- Is benign.

Diagnosis

- It should be excised for histopathological examination;
- Vanillyl mandelic acid and alpha-fetoprotein serum levels are raised.

Management

Excision for diagnostic reasons. It may recur.

Melkersson–Rosenthal syndrome

Melkersson–Rosenthal syndrome consists of lower motor neurone facial paralysis, facial oedema, fissured tongue and plicated mucosal swelling. Not all patients have every component of the syndrome, which is closely related to orofacial granulomatosis and oral Crohn's disease.

Mucocoele

See Chapter 5

Mucormycosis (zygomycosis; phycomycosis)

Definition

A deep mycosis caused by *Mucor* and *Rhizopus* fungi of the order Mucorales (of the class Zygomycetes)

Incidence

Uncommon

Age mainly affected

Adults

Sex mainly affected

M=F

Aetiology

The fungi causing mucormycosis (mucoraceae) are ubiquitous worldwide in soil, manure and decaying organic matter, and infection is found worldwide. Mucoraceae can commonly be cultured from the nose, throat, mouth and faeces of many healthy individuals. Disease is seen in immunocompromised persons.

Clinical features

- Disease is virtually unheard of in otherwise healthy individuals.
- In immunocompromising conditions such as leukaemia, lymphoma, diabetes with ketoacidosis, burns, malnutrition, cancer chemotherapy, immunosuppressive therapy and HIV disease, there can be rhinocerebral zygomycosis, which typically:
  - Commences in the nasal cavity or paranasal sinuses;
  - Causes pain and nasal discharge, and fever;
  - May then invade the palate and invade intracranially. Zygomycosis still has a mortality approaching 20%.

Diagnosis

- Radiography; typically shows thickening of the antral mucosa with patchy destruction of the walls;
- MRI or CT may help;
- Smear;
- Biopsy.

Management

- Control underlying disease;
- Surgical debridement;
- Systemic amphotericin (Table 10.8).

Mucosal neuromas

Familial syndromes of multiple endocrine neoplasia (MEN) occur in at least three separate clinical patterns, MEN types 1, 2a and 2b(3).

MEN type 2b (3 or Sipple syndrome) is an autosomal dominant syndrome carried on chromosome 10, characterized by multiple neuromas that are actually mucosal, and submucosal hamartomatous proliferations of nerve axons, Schwann cells and ganglion cells.

Most patients have the following:

- Thickened eyelids and conjunctivae, with multiple neuromas producing an irregular lumpy appearance;
- An asthenic Marfanoid habitus, with high arched palate, pectus excavatum, arachnodactyly and kyphoscoliosis, but without the lens subluxation and cardiovascular abnormalities of Marfan's syndrome;
- Thick, slightly everted lips with a bumpy surface due to the multiple neuromas especially affecting the upper lip;
- Neuromas in the tongue, mainly anteriorly, and commissures but less commonly on the buccal mucosa, rare on the gingivae or palate;
- The inferior dental canal may be widened;
- Neuromatosis throughout the gastrointestinal tract, which may result in constipation or megacolon;
- Endocrinopathies; medullary thyroid carcinoma (80%), phaeochromocytoma (30%) and parathyroid hyperplasia.

Diagnosis

- Clinical;
- Urinary levels of vanillyl mandelic acid and calcitonin (raised);
- Scan thyroid and adrenals.

Management

Prophylactic thyroidectomy

Mucositis

Mucositis is common after irradiation of tumours of the head and neck, if the radiation field involves the oral mucosa. Arising within 3 weeks of the irradiation, there is generalized erythema, and sometimes ulceration (Figures 4.58 and 4.143). There is no specific treatment (see page 107) but oral hygiene should be improved and potent analgesics given (Tables 10.1 and 10.2).

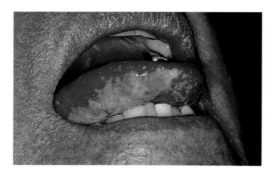

Figure 4.143
Mucositis following radiotherapy

Myxoma

This is rare in the oral cavity. It can arise in bone or soft tissue and is aggressive and difficult to eradicate because of its tendency to infiltrate normal tissue.

Naevi (pigmented)

Definition

Congenital, usually hyperpigmented, lesion

Incidence

Common

Age mainly affected

Any

Sex mainly affected

M=F

Aetiology

Genetic. Some are seen in autosomal dominant conditions such as NAME (**n**aevi, **a**trial myxoma, **m**yxoid neurofibroma, **e**phelides) or LAMB (**l**entigines, **a**trial myxoma, **m**ultiple **b**lue naevi) syndromes.

Clinical features

Naevi:

- Are seen particularly on the vermilion border of the lips, the gingivae and hard palate (Figure 4.144);
- Are usually grey, brown or bluish macules (Figure 4.145);
- Are typically asymptomatic;
- Are usually <1 cm across;
- Do not change rapidly in size or colour;
- Are usually benign, but the malignant potential is uncertain.

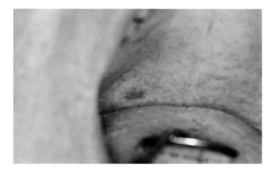

Figure 4.144
Naevus in a common site

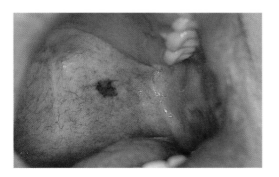

Figure 4.145
Naevus

Diagnosis

Biopsy is invariably indicated to exclude melanoma (both are HMB–45 positive).

The terminology relating to naevi can be somewhat confusing. *Melanocytes* are pigment-producing cells characterized by the ability to synthesize via the enzyme dihydroxyphenylalanine (DOPA). A group of melanocytes (generally four or more) in contact with the basal layer of the epithelium but budding downwards into the lamina propria, is termed a *theque*. Clinical and histopathological terms include the following:

Intramucosal naevus

A cellular naevus in which there is little or no abnormality of melanocytes in the epithelium. The main feature is the presence of packets of naevus cells with few mitoses in the lamina propria. Such naevi may be clinically nonpigmented but are typically brown or black, macular or slightly raised and very slow growing. This is the common naevus, 50% of all oral naevi, and is benign. It is rare on the tongue.

Junctional naevus

This is clinically indistinguishable from the intramucosal naevus but biopsy shows theques of melanocytes at the epitheliomesenchymal junction. It is rare but may represent a premalignant state.

Compound naevus

This is clinically indistinguishable from the intramucosal naevus, but biopsy shows a pigmented or cellular naevus in which the histological features include both junctional activity and the presence of naevus cells in the lamina propria. It appears in the teens and may have some malignant potential.

Blue naevus

This is typically a bluish papule or macule at the junction of hard and soft palate. The pigment-producing cells are fusiform or spindle-shaped and found within the connective tissue. It is benign and accounts for about 25% of oral naevi.

Freckle (ephelis)

An area of increased melanin pigmentation. Result of functionally overactive melanocytes: no other histological changes. Lesions are stimulated by ultraviolet irradiation.

Lentigo

An area of increased melanin pigmentation which shows histologically a linear replacement of keratinocytes in the basal layer of the epithelium by melanocytes. This replacement does not reach the level of theque formation.

Management

Excision biopsy is recommended mainly to exclude malignancy, and also because of the malignant potential of some, particularly the junctional naevus, and for cosmetic reasons.

Neurilemoma

Neurilemoma or Schwannoma arises from Schwann cells usually in the 3rd to 5th decade as a slow-growing firm swelling, typically in the tongue. It should be excised.

Neurofibroma

Neurofibroma is a rare lesion which typically affects the tongue. It represents a benign overgrowth of all elements of a peripheral nerve (axon cylinder, Schwann cells and fibrous connective tissue), arranged in a variety of patterns. Neurofibromas may occur singly, especially in the tongue, or multiply as a feature of MEN 2b (page 191) neurofibromatosis (von Recklinghausen's disease) and then rarely may undergo sarcomatous change. Neurofibromas should be excised if symptomatic.

Neutropenias

Neutropenias predispose to rapidly destructive periodontal disease and to oral ulceration.

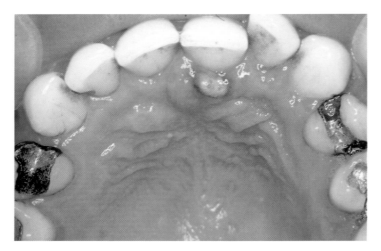

Figure 4.146
Cyclic neutropenia producing ulcers at the gingival margin

Cyclic neutropenia is a rare form which produces a drop in polymorphonuclear neutrophil count, and sometimes other leukocytes, about every 21 days. Destructive periodontal disease, recurrent ulcerative gingivitis and recurrent mouth ulcers (Figures 4.66 and 4.146) are frequent manifestations (see page 119).

Oral submucous fibrosis

Definition

Submucous fibrosis is a condition characterized by fibrosis of the oral submucosa only.

Incidence

Uncommon

Age mainly affected

Adults from the Indian subcontinent

Sex mainly affected

F>M

Aetiology

Oral submucous fibrosis (OSMF) appears to be caused by exposure to the areca nut. It is found virtually exclusively in persons from the Indian continent. Betel (areca) nut chewing, possibly affects collagen cross-linking via copper.

Clinical features

- In the early stages OSMF may be symptomless;
- A burning sensation with vesiculation and then erosions in the palate and/or tongue are the earliest features;
- Tight vertical bands in buccal mucosa (or palate or tongue) may progress to severely restricted oral opening (Figure 4.147);
- Symmetrical fibrosis of the cheeks, lips or palate can be so severe that the affected site becomes white and firm;
- Areas appear almost white but unlike leukoplakia the mucosa is typically smooth, thin and atrophic, and the pallor is due to underlying fibrosis and ischaemia, and is symmetrically distributed;
- The oral mucosa is affected mainly although oesophageal involvement may occur;
- Often anaemia is present;
- Taste may also be impaired;
- The epithelium may show dysplasia in about 15%, and carcinoma may develop in up to 5% of patients with submucous fibrosis in a 10-year period.

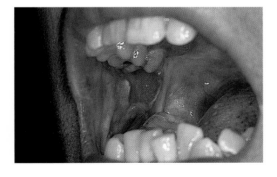

Figure 4.147
Oral submucous fibrosis

Diagnosis

The diagnosis is essentially clinical; only scleroderma and scarring from other causes are likely to confuse the diagnosis. However, biopsy and haematology may be required, particularly if dysplasia or carcinoma are suspected.

Management

The use of areca nut should be abandoned.

- Asymptomatic lesions should be observed only;
- Symptomatic lesions are very difficult to deal with.

Exercises, intralesional corticosteroids, interferon and surgery have all been tried with limited success.

Orofacial granulomatosis

Definition

The term orofacial granulomatosis (OFG) has been introduced for oral granulomatous reactions that are not associated with any detectable systemic disease or foreign bodies.

Incidence

Uncommon

Age mainly affected

From childhood

Sex mainly affected

M=F

Aetiology

In some patients the reaction is to common food and drink additives such as cinnamon or tartrazine or benzoates; others have a postulated reaction to food or other antigens such as paratuberculosis.

Clinical features

General features of Crohn's disease (abdominal pain, persistent diarrhoea with passage of blood and mucus, anaemia and weight loss) and of sarcoidosis (weakness, dyspnoea, lymphadenopathy) are absent in OFG. Features of OFG may include, in any combination:

- Facial and/or labial swelling (Figures 4.148 and 4.149);
- Angular stomatitis and/or cracked lips;
- Ulcers;
- Mucosal tags and/or cobble-stoning (Figure 4.150);

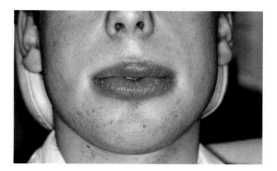

Figure 4.148
Orofacial granulomatosis: facial swelling

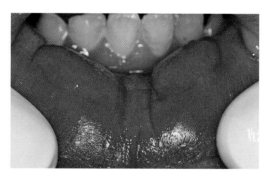

Figure 4.149
Orofacial granulomatosis: labial swelling

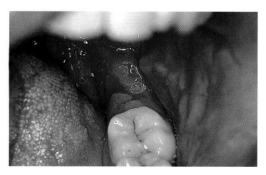

Figure 4.150
Orofacial granulomatosis: mucosal tags

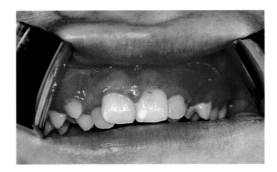

Figure 4.151
Orofacial granulomatosis: gingival lesions

- Gingival swelling (Figure 4.151);
- Cervical lymph node enlargement;
- Rarely, acrodermatitis enteropathica.

Miescher's cheilitis is where lip swelling is seen in isolation.
Melkersson–Rosenthal syndrome is where lip or facial swelling is seen with fissured tongue and/or facial palsy.

Diagnosis

- An oral biopsy may confirm the presence of lymphoedema and granulomas, suggestive of one of the conditions, but cannot reliably differentiate OFG from Crohn's disease or sarcoidosis;
- Dietary-related cases of OFG can only be confirmed by an exclusion diet to eliminate food allergens. Skin tests may be useful;
- Blood tests, and intestinal radiology, endoscopy and biopsy may be required to exclude gastrointestinal lesions of Crohn's disease;
- Chest radiography, serum levels of calcium, angiotensin-converting enzyme (SACE), gallium scan and biopsy may be needed to exclude sarcoidosis.

Management

- An exclusion diet should be tried;
- Intralesional corticosteroids may help control oral lesions such as swelling; occasionally systemic sulphasalazine or other agents are required (Table 10.6).

Regular follow-up should be maintained to ensure that systemic disease is recognized at an early stage. Some patients with apparent

OFG do actually have latent systemic disease such as Crohn's disease or sarcoidosis which develops months or years later, but many others remain apparently otherwise healthy.

Pachyonychia congenita

This is a rare autosomal dominant disorder seen especially in Jews and Slavs, characterized by:

- Oral white lesions; by 10 years most have white lesions on the lateral tongue and buccal mucosae (Jadassohn–Lewandowsky syndrome). Some do not and are then termed Jackson–Lawler syndrome;
- Natal teeth may be seen;
- Nail defects; yellow thickened;
- Skin thickening;
- Abnormal hair and cornea;
- Palmoplantar hyperkeratosis and hyperhidrosis.

There is no predisposition to malignancy.

Papilloma

Definition

This is a benign neoplasm of epithelium with an anemone-like appearance.

Incidence

Uncommon

Age mainly affected

Adults

Sex mainly affected

M=F

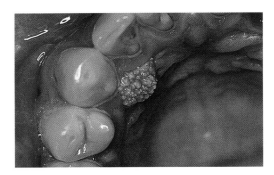

Figure 4.152
Papilloma

Aetiology

Many are caused by human papillomaviruses (HPV): usually HPV 6 or 11.

Clinical features

Papillomas are far more common than warts in the oral cavity. Most:

- Are cauliflower-like lesions with a whitish colour;
- Are <1 cm in diameter;
- Are seen at the junction of the hard and soft palate (Figures 4.152 and 9.35). The lips, gingiva or tongue may occasionally be affected;
- Appear to be and remain benign, unlike papillomas of the larynx or bowel, which may undergo malignant transformation.

Diagnosis and management

Oral papillomas should be removed and examined histologically to establish a correct diagnosis. Excision must be total, deep and wide enough to include any abnormal cells beyond the zone of the pedicle. Some use topical podophyllin but this is potentially teratogenic and toxic to brain, kidney and myocardium.

Paracoccidioidomycosis (South American blastomycosis)

Definition

A deep mycosis caused by *Paracoccidioides brasiliensis*

Incidence

Uncommon. Found mainly in Latin America, especially in Brazil, and also in Colombia, Venezuela, Uruguay and Argentina.

Age mainly affected

Adults

Sex mainly affected

M=F

Aetiology

Spores are presumably inhaled.

Clinical features

Subclinical infection is not uncommon in endemic areas. Clinical paracoccidioidomycosis commonly presents as chronic pulmonary disease, with cough, dyspnoea, fever, weight loss and haemoptysis. Oral lesions, which are chronic, are often granular or exophytic and ulcerated.

Diagnosis

- Smear;
- Biopsy;
- Culture can also be diagnostically useful, but *P. brasiliensis* grows only extremely slowly.

Management

Systemic amphotericin, ketoconazole, miconazole, fluconazole or itraconazole (Table 10.8)

Pemphigoid

Definition

Pemphigoid is the term given to a group of autoimmune disorders in which there is subepithelial vesiculation.

Incidence

Uncommon

Age mainly affected

Middle-aged and elderly

Sex mainly affected

F>M

Aetiology

Mainly autoimmune, resulting from damage to the attachment of the epithelial basement membrane, caused by autoantibodies against various proteins of the membrane especially integrins. A very few cases are drug-induced (e.g. by frusemide or penicillamine) (Figures 4.153–4.156).

Clinical features

Mucous membrane pemphigoid (MMP) is the main variant that presents with oral manifestations. The oral lesions of MMP affect especially the gingivae and palate, but rarely the vermilion, and may include the following:

- Desquamative gingivitis. This is one of the main manifestations, and MMP is one of the most common causes of this complaint (Figure 4.157). The gingivitis is typically rather patchy. There is usually persistent soreness but some cases are asymptomatic;
- Bullae or vesicles which are tense (Figure 4.158), may be blood-filled and remain intact for several days. Pressure on the blister may cause it to spread;
- Persistent irregular erosions or ulcers after the blisters burst (Figure 4.159). Typically these are covered with a yellowish fibrinous slough and have surrounding erythema, and thus resemble erosive lichen planus except that no white lesions are present in MMP;
- Scarring, rarely.

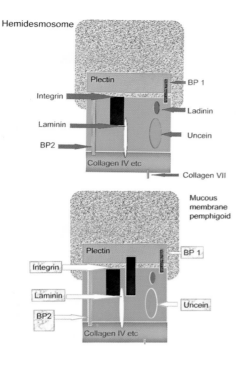

Figure 4.153
Hemidesmosome and basement membrane zone structure

Figure 4.154
Pemphigoid: antigens to which autoantibodies are directed in various forms of mucous membrane pemphigoid

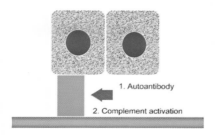

Figure 4.155
Pemphigoid: immunopathogenesis

Figure 4.156
Pemphigoid: immunostaining

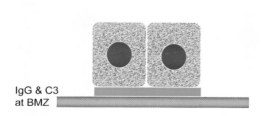

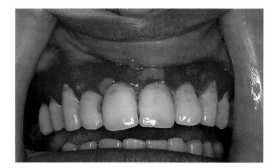

Figure 4.157
Pemphigoid causing desquamative gingivitis

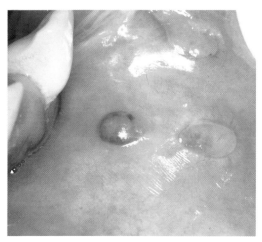

Figure 4.158
Pemphigoid: blisters

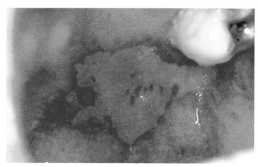

Figure 4.159
Pemphigoid: chronic erosions

MMP may also cause:

- Conjunctival scarring (entropion, symblepharon or ankyloble-pharon; Figure 4.160); or glaucoma leading to impaired sight;
- Laryngeal scarring which may lead to stenosis;
- Skin blisters rarely.

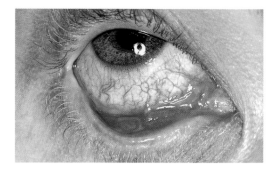

Figure 4.160
*Pemphigoid with
conjunctival lesions and
symblepharon*

Diagnosis

- The history and clinical appearances are often suggestive of MMP but cannot reliably differentiate from other vesiculobullous disorders;
- Biopsy (including immunostaining) is essential and usually shows subepithelial vesiculation with linear deposits of IgG and sometimes C3 at the basement membrane zone. Lesions showing IgA deposits as well are usually resistant to treatment;
- An ophthalmological opinion is always indicated.

Management

- Oral hygiene should be improved (Tables 10.1 and 10.2);
- Symptomatic patients often respond to corticosteroids, but these may need to be potent topical agents such as fluocinolone acetonide cream used for 5 minutes twice daily, or in a vacuum-formed splint at night for the treatment of desquamative gingivitis;
- Rarely, systemic corticosteroids or dapsone are indicated for recalcitrant lesions (Table 10.7).

Pemphigus

Definition

Pemphigus is an autoimmune disease with antibodies directed against the glycoprotein coat of epidermal and mucosal cells, which separate, forming thin-rooted blisters within the epithelium (acantholysis or intraepithelial vesiculation).

Incidence

Rare

Age mainly affected

Middle-aged and elderly

Sex mainly affected

F>M

Aetiology

Pemphigus is an autoimmune disorder with antibodies directed against proteins of the desmosomes that are responsible for cell–cell adhesion (intercellular cement) in stratified squamous epithelium. The most common form, pemphigus vulgaris, is related to antibodies against desmoglein 3 (Figures 4.161–4.164).

Pemphigus vulgaris has a predilection for Arabs, Jews and others originating from the Mediterranean area, Asians, and an association with HLA-DR4 and HLA-DR6. Rare cases are related to neoplasia (paraneoplastic pemphigus), garlic or drugs (Tables 4.12 and 4.13), or are infective (fogo selvagem in Brazil).

Table 4.12   Neoplasms associated with paraneoplastic pemphigus

Non-Hodgkin's lymphoma
Leukaemia
Waldenstrom's macroglobulinaemia
Castleman's tumour
Thymoma
Spindle cell neoplasms

Table 4.13   Drugs inducing pemphigus

Captopril
Mercaptopropionyl glycine
Penicillamine
Penicillins
Piroxicam
Pyritinol
Rifampicin
5-Thiopyridoxine
Thiopronine

Desmosome

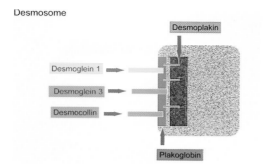

Figure 4.161
Structure of desmosome

Pemphigus vulgaris

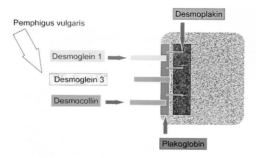

Figure 4.162
Pemphigus vulgaris: autoantibody is directed against desmoglein 3 in pemphigus vulgaris

1
IgG antibody to desmoglein

2
Antibody binds to desmosomes

3
Plasminogen activation ➡ plasmin

4   ACANTHOLYSIS

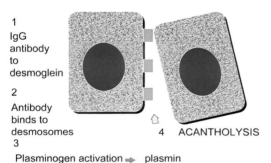

Figure 4.163
Pemphigus: sequence of immunological and other changes

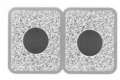

IgG & C3 intercellularly

Figure 4.164
Pemphigus: immunostaining shows intercellular deposits of IgG and C_3

Clinical features

The oral mucosa are affected in 95% of patients with pemphigus vulgaris and may be the initial presentation of the disease in 50%. Pressure on the blister may cause it to spread (Nikolsky sign). Oral lesions include the following:

- Bullae, which rapidly break down to produce persistent irregular ragged-edged erosions or ulcers (Figure 4.165);
- The partial loss of the epithelium tends initially to leave red erosions with a surrounding whitish area due to necrotic epithelium, but when there is secondary infection a full thickness ulcer with a fibrinous slough results.

Lesions are seen especially where there is trauma, such as on the palate (Figure 4.166). Lesions are rare in the floor of the mouth.

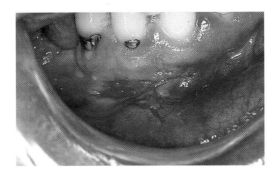

Figure 4.165
Pemphigus: irregular erosion

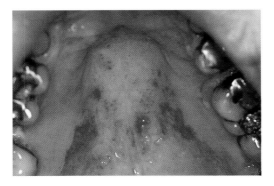

Figure 4.166
Pemphigus: irregular chronic erosions

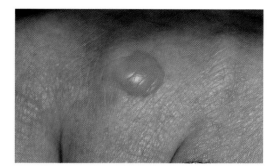

Figure 4.167
Pemphigus: skin blister

Lesions may also affect:

- Skin, as large flaccid blisters, seen especially where there is trauma (Figure 4.167);
- Other mucous membranes, especially ocular, nasal and genital.

Paraneoplastic pemphigus differs somewhat in that it:

- Typically affects the lips with erosions and may resemble erythema multiforme;
- Presents with skin lesions that can mimic erythema multiforme, pemphigoid or lichen planus.

Diagnosis

- A biopsy (with immunostaining) is essential. Acantholysis and/or intercellular deposition of IgG and sometimes C3 in a wire-netting pattern are typical of pemphigus vulgaris;
- Serum antibodies to epithelial intercellular cement should be sought as they may show some relationship to disease activity.

Management

- Neoplasia, drugs and other autoimmune disorders should be excluded;
- Immunosuppressive agents are required since this is a life-threatening condition;
- High-dose systemic corticosteroids with steroid-sparing agents such as azathioprine, levamisole, dapsone or gold are indicated (Table 10.7);

- Oral lesions are persistent, and are often recalcitrant even when cutaneous lesions are controlled by treatment. Topical cortico-steroids may help (Table 10.6);
- Oral hygiene should be improved (Tables 10.1 and 10.2).

Peutz–Jeghers syndrome

Definition

Peutz–Jeghers syndrome is as an inherited trait characterized by hamartomatous intestinal polyposis and mucocutaneous melanotic pigmentation especially circumorally.

Incidence

Rare

Age mainly affected

From birth

Sex mainly affected

M=F

Aetiology

Autosomal dominant

Clinical features

- Pigmented oral and perioral macules. Discrete, brown to bluish black macules are seen mainly around the oral, nasal and ocular orifices. The lips, especially the lower, have pigmented macules in about 98% of patients. The skin lesions, but not the oral ones, tend to fade with age;

- Intestinal polyps mainly in the small intestine, which may rarely:
  - Undergo malignant change;
  - Produce intussusception.
- Increased risk of carcinomas of gastrointestinal tract, pancreas, breast and reproductive organs.

Diagnosis and management

The diagnosis is clinical. Patients should receive close follow-up by a physician.

Pigmented naevi

See Naevi

Precancerous lesions and conditions

These are not a single clinical entity but several can predispose to malignancy; they are better termed 'potentially' malignant. They include:

- Erythroplasia;
- Oral submucous fibrosis;
- Actinic cheilitis;
- Discoid lupus erythematosus;
- Chronic hyperplastic candidosis;
- Some leukoplakias;
- Some lichen planus;
- Syphilitic glossitis;
- Atypia in immunocompromised patients.

Proliferative verrucous leukoplakia

This is a rapidly growing nodular leukoplakia seen mainly in elderly tobacco-users, especially females, often associated with papillomavirus, and with a high predisposition to malignant change.

Pseudocarcinomatous hyperplasia (pseudoepitheliomatous hyperplasia)

This is not a clinical condition, but several entities can exhibit histological features which, to the untrained eye, can mimic carcinoma. They include:

- Blastomycoses;
- Chronic trauma;
- Discoid lupus erythematosus;
- Granular cell tumour;
- Median rhomboid glossitis;
- Necrotizing sialometaplasia;
- Pemphigus vegetans.

Pyogenic granuloma

Definition

This is a proliferative, painless red and friable reactive vascular lesion, which bleeds readily. It is not actually a granuloma.

Incidence

Uncommon

Age mainly affected

Young adults

Sex mainly affected

F>M

Aetiology

The pyogenic granuloma (lobular capillary haemangioma) appears to represent an excessive reaction to trauma or infection. Many arise in response to irritation from dental plaque on:

- Calculus;
- A dental restoration;
- A prosthesis.

Pregnancy and bone marrow transplantation appear to predispose to pyogenic granulomas.

Clinical features

The head and neck region, especially the lip (Figure 4.168), is a common location for pyogenic granuloma and for the related intravascular papillary endothelial hyperplasia (IPEH, Masson's haemangioma or pseudoangiosarcoma).
  Pyogenic granuloma usually:

- Is an exophytic ulcerated lump, red in colour;
- Bleeds readily if traumatized;
- Affects sites that are traumatized such as the lip, gingiva (especially the maxillary anterior labial), buccal mucosa at the occlusal line or tongue;
- May grow to 1 cm or more in diameter.

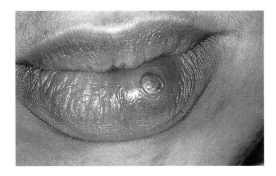

Figure 4.168
Pyogenic granuloma

Diagnosis and management

These benign lesions should be excised but will readily recur if excision is not adequate. There is no granuloma formation, rather there is granulation tissue. Benign atypical vascular lesions, such as IPEH, may exhibit cytological or architectural features that simulate angiosarcoma so that considerable caution is required.

Pyostomatitis vegetans

Definition

Pustules and ulcers in the mouth, related to inflammatory bowel disease

Incidence

Rare

Age mainly affected

Adults

Sex mainly affected

M=F

Aetiology

Less than 50 cases have been recorded and most patients have had ulcerative colitis or Crohn's disease. Some have had liver disease.

Clinical features

Oral lesions termed pyostomatitis vegetans are seen especially on the gingivae and palate, rarely on the tongue and include:

- Deep fissures;
- Pustules;
- Ulcers (Figure 4.169);
- Papillary projections.

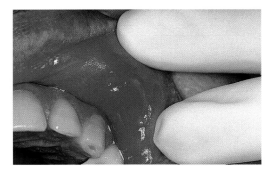

Figure 4.169
Pyostomatitis vegetans can produce snail-track ulcers similar to those seen in secondary syphilis

The course of these lesions tends to follow that of the bowel disease. Patients may also have lesions on:

- Skin;
- Genitals.

Diagnosis

- Oral lesional biopsy;
- Haematology; eosinophilia common;
- Gastrointestinal investigations.

Management

Salazopyrine or systemic corticosteroids

Racial pigmentation

There is no direct correlation between skin colour and oral pigmentation. The most usual cause of brown oral mucosal pigmentation is ethnic: it occurs in Blacks and Asians and also in patients of Mediterranean descent. The pigmentation is usually symmetrically distributed over the anterior gingiva and palatal mucosa (Figures 4.170–4.172) but may be seen elsewhere. Pigmentation may be first noted by the patient in adult life and then incorrectly assumed to be acquired rather than congenital in origin.

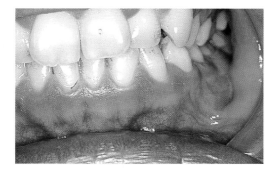

Figure 4.170
Racial pigmentation

Radiotherapy-induced lesions

Mucositis, xerostomia and loss of taste are almost invariable after irradiation involving the oral region, though the severity is often related to the

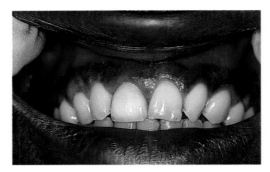

Figure 4.171
Racial pigmentation

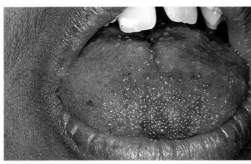

Figure 4.172
Racial pigmentation

dose of radiotherapy used. Infections (caries, candidiasis, acute sialadeni-tis) and dental hypersensitivity are mainly secondary to reduced salivary function. Osteoradionecrosis, osteomyelitis and trismus are secondary to endarteritis of the small arteries in bone and muscle. Radiotherapy involving the jaws may well affect tooth and root development, produc-ing results similar to those seen in patients on chemotherapy.

Recurrent aphthous stomatitis

See Aphthae

Sarcoidosis

Definition

Sarcoidosis is a chronic disease of unknown cause, in which granulo-mas form particularly in the lungs, lymph nodes (especially the hilar nodes), salivary glands and other sites such as the mouth.

Incidence
Uncommon, seen mainly in black patients

Age mainly affected
Adult

Sex mainly affected
F>M

Aetiology
Unknown: an infectious aetiology has been suggested but not proven.

Clinical features
Sarcoidosis is protean in its manifestations and can involve virtually any tissue. It typically causes:

- Bilateral hilar lymphadenopathy;
- Pulmonary infiltration;
- Skin;
- Erythema nodosum;
- Lymphadenopathy;
- Lung involvement;
- Eye lesions.

Orofacial features include:

- Cervical lymphadenopathy;
- Enlarged salivary glands occasionally. Heerfordt's syndrome (salivary and lachrymal swelling, facial palsy and uveitis) is rare;
- Xerostomia;
- Mucosal nodules;
- Gingival hyperplasia;
- Labial swelling.

Diagnosis
- Biopsy of affected tissue shows characteristic granulomas that are noncaseating, contain multinucleated giant cells and are surrounded by lymphocytes. They must be differentiated from tuberculosis, Crohn's disease, OFG and various foreign body reactions. In over 50% of patients with bilateral hilar lymphadenopathy, biopsy of a labial salivary gland shows typical granulomas;

- Lymphadenopathy can be confirmed by chest radiography (showing hilar lymphadenopathy);
- Gallium is taken up by macrophages in the granulomas; a scan may show uptake in involved lymph nodes, salivary and lachrymal glands;
- The Kveim test is positive in about 80% of patients with sarcoidosis. The test used to be carried out by an intracutaneous injection of a heat-sterilized suspension of human lymphoid tissue affected with sarcoidosis. After 4–6 weeks the area was biopsied and, if positive, showed well-formed epithelioid noncaseating granulomas;
- Assay of serum angiotensin converting enzyme (SACE) and adenosine deaminase levels (both raised) have now superseded the Kveim test;
- Serum calcium levels are often raised.

Management

- Patients with only minor symptoms of sarcoidosis often require no treatment. The condition can be self-limiting;
- Corticosteroids are used if there is active disease of the lungs or eyes, cerebral involvement, or other serious complications such as hypercalcaemia.

Scleroderma

Definition

A generalized condition in which normal connective tissue is replaced by dense collagen

Incidence

Rare

Age mainly affected

Middle-aged and elderly

Sex mainly affected

F>M

Aetiology

Unknown, probably autoimmune. A localized form, morphoea, may be related to infection with *Borrelia burgdorferi*.

Clinical features

- Skin tight and waxy;
- Raynaud's syndrome (finger vasoconstriction on cooling);
- Perioral radial folds (Mona Lisa face);
- Oral opening restricted with microstomia (Figure 4.173);
- Pale fibrotic 'chicken' tongue;
- Frenulum sclerosis, especially in those with gastrointestinal involvement;
- Widened periodontal space on radiography in a few, but teeth do not become mobile;
- Telangiectasia;
- Bone lesions;
- Secondary Sjögren's syndrome;
- Dysphagia.

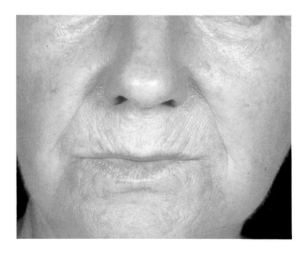

Figure 4.173
Scleroderma

Rare variants:

- CRST syndrome (**c**alcinosis, **R**aynaud's syndrome, **s**clerodactyly, **t**elangiectasia); CREST includes oesophageal lesions;
- Thibierge–Weissenbach syndrome (widespread internal calcification).

Diagnosis

- Clinical features;
- Histopathology;
- Auto-antibodies (ANF and Scl 70 especially);
- Oral lesions: differentiate from OSMF, telangiectasia (e.g. HHT) and secondary Sjögren's syndrome.

Management

Penicillamine

Self-mutilation

Factitious or artefactual lesions are seen in some patients with the following:

- Learning disability (Figures 1.26, 1.30 and 4.174);
- Munchausen's syndrome (deliberate seeking of medical/surgical intervention);
- Psychiatric disease;
- Sensory loss in the area, as in neuropathies, Lesch–Nyhan syndrome (sex-linked hyperuricaemia), Gilles de la Tourette syndrome (tic, coprolalia and copropraxia), congenital indifference to pain or familial dysautonomia (Riley–Day syndrome).

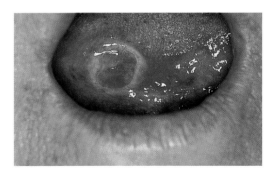

Figure 4.174
Self-induced (factitious) injury showing ulceration with a keratotic margin

Smoker's melanosis

Irregular hyperpigmented macules especially on the maxillary anterior labial gingivae, especially interdentally. They may also be seen

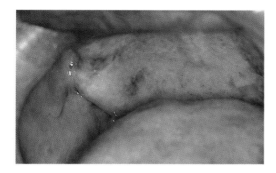

Figure 4.175
Smokers' pigmentation

in the buccal mucosa, floor of mouth and soft palate mucosa, especially in heavy smokers and in females (Figure 4.175). These lesions often abate if smoking is stopped.

Stomatitis medicamentosa

Oral ulceration may be induced by a number of drugs, by a range of different mechanisms. In some, there may also be cutaneous lesions or lesions of other mucosae. Drugs particularly implicated include:

- Antibiotics;
- Non-steroidal anti-inflammatory drugs (NSAIDs);
- Anticonvulsants;
- Antihypertensives;
- Antidepressants.

A careful drug history is required; the offending agent should be stopped.

Sturge–Weber syndrome (encephalofacial angiomatosis)

This is a neuroectodermal disorder in which an orofacial haemangioma often appears to be limited to the area of distribution of one or more of the divisions of the trigeminal nerve. The angioma affects part of the face and usually extends into the occipital lobe of the brain. The haemangioma may extend intraorally and be associated with hypertrophy of the affected jaw, macrodontia and accelerated tooth eruption (Figure 4.176). Radiography shows intracranial calcification of the angioma. This produces epilepsy and often hemiplegia and results in learning disability.

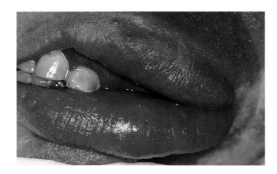

Figure 4.176
Sturge–Weber syndrome

Submucous fibrosis

See page 196

Syphilis

Definition

This is a systemic sexually transmitted infection with *Treponema pallidum* that can affect the genitals, skin, cardiovascular and neurological systems in particular.

Incidence

Uncommon, but increasing dramatically, and seen mainly in adults who are sexually promiscuous such as some:

- Prostitutes;
- Intravenous drug users;
- Promiscuous men who have sex with men;
- Business travellers;
- Members of the armed services.

Age mainly affected

Adult

Sex mainly affected

M>F

Aetiology

Treponema pallidum

Clinical features

Primary syphilis (Hunterian or hard chancre)

The incubation period of 9–90 days is followed by regional lymphadenitis and a small papule which develops into a large painless indurated ulcer (chancre), which heals spontaneously in 1–2 months. Rarely chancres are seen on the lip (upper) or intraorally, usually on the tongue.

Secondary syphilis

- Oral lesions (mucous patches, split papules or snail-track ulcers) (Figure 4.177) are highly infectious. They are seen mainly on the tongue;
- Coppery coloured rash typically on palms and soles;
- Condylomata lata or spilt papules;
- Generalized lymph node enlargement can also be present.

Tertiary syphilis

Oral lesions, which are noninfectious, may include:

- Glossitis (leukoplakia);
- Gumma (usually midline in palate or tongue).

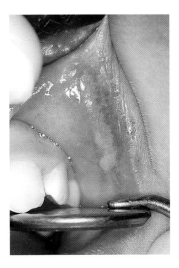

Figure 4.177
Syphilis

These may be associated with:

- Cardiovascular complications (aortic aneurysm); or
- Neurosyphilis (tabes dorsalis; general paralysis of the insane; Argyll–Robinson pupils).

Diagnosis

T. pallidum may be detected in a lesional smear by dark-field examination. Serology is positive from late in the primary stage. Specialist referral is indicated, and contact tracing will be required.

Management

Penicillin (by depot injection) is required or, if the patient is allergic to penicillin, erythromycin or tetracycline.

Thrombocytopathy

Spontaneous gingival bleeding is often an early feature in platelet deficiencies or defects. Postextraction bleeding may be a problem. Oral petechiae and ecchymoses appear mainly at sites of trauma but can be spontaneous. Petechiae appear therefore, mainly in the buccal mucosa, on the lateral margin of the tongue, and at the junction of hard and soft palates. Petechiae and ecchymoses also appear readily on the skin, especially if there is trauma. Even the pressure from a sphygmomanometer can cause petechiae during the measurement of blood pressure.

Transplantation patients

Oral complications are common and can be a major cause of morbidity following organ transplantation, especially bone marrow transplantation (BMT), from the effects of the underlying disease, chemo- or radiotherapy, and, in BMT, from graft-versus-host disease (GVHD).

The oral manifestations of acute GVHD have not been well documented but consist of the following:

- Small white lesions affect the buccal and lingual mucosa early on, but clear by day 14;

- Erythema and ulceration, most pronounced at 7–11 days after BMT, and may be associated with obvious infection. The ventrum of the tongue, buccal and labial mucosa, and gingiva may be affected by ulceration or mucositis;
- Cheilitis;
- Lichenoid plaques or striae;
- Infections; candidiasis is common, as is herpes simplex stomatitis (occasionally zoster);
- Oral purpura.

The oral lesions in chronic GVHD are coincident with skin lesions, and include the following:

- Generalized mucosal erythema;
- Lichenoid lesions, mainly in the buccal mucosa;
- Xerostomia; most significant in the first 14 days after transplantation and a consequence of drug treatment, irradiation and/or GVHD;
- Infections; especially candidiasis;
- Hairy leukoplakia;
- Cyclosporin may induce gingival hyperplasia.

The main complications in organ transplants include:

- Infections, especially candidiasis;
- Cyclosporin-induced gingival hyperplasia;
- Predisposition to leukoplakia, hairy leukoplakia and some malignant tumours such as lip carcinoma, lymphomas, and Kaposi's sarcoma.

Tuberculosis (TB)

Definition

This is mainly a mycobacterial infection resulting in caseating granuloma formation and scarring.

Incidence

One-third of the world's population is infected with TB, but it is uncommon in the developed world. It is seen there especially in:

- Vagrants;
- Intravenous drug users;
- Alcoholics;
- Immigrant persons from the developing world;
- HIV-infected persons.

Age mainly affected

Middle-aged and elderly

Sex mainly affected

M>F

Aetiology

- Mycobacteria: typically *M. tuberculosis*, usually contracted from infected sputum, sometimes (*M. bovis*) from infected milk.
- Increasingly, but still rarely, atypical mycobacteria (nontuberculous mycobacteria: NTM), such as *M. avium-intracellulare* (MAI), *M. scrofulaceum* or *M. kansasii*, are involved—especially in HIV infection.

Clinical features

Tuberculosis is often a multisystem infection which primarily affects:

- Lungs;
- Bones.

Mouth ulceration is rarely detected and usually presents as a single chronic ulcer on the dorsum of the tongue associated with (postprimary) pulmonary infection (Figure 4.178). Lymph-node enlargement may be a presenting feature of TB or NTM infection.

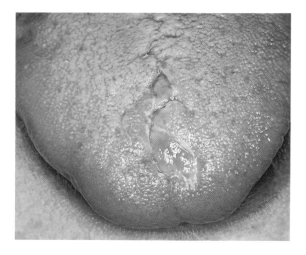

Figure 4.178
Tuberculosis: ulceration on the dorsum of the tongue may be seen in pulmonary TB

Diagnosis

Specialist referral is indicated. Biopsy, sputum culture, chest radiography and other investigations may be indicated.

Management

Combination chemotherapy is required. TB is increasingly multidrug resistant in HIV-infected persons.

Tuberose sclerosis (see page 298)

Ulcerative colitis

Definition

Ulcerative colitis is an inflammatory bowel disease with ulcers and polyps (which may undergo malignant change) in the colon.

Incidence

Uncommon

Age mainly affected

Middle-aged and elderly

Sex mainly affected

M=F

Aetiology

Unknown

Clinical features

General features may include:

- Persistent diarrhoea, frequently painless with passage of blood and mucus in severe cases;

- Iron-deficiency anaemia;
- Weight loss.

Oral features may include:

- Irregular chronic ulcers;
- Mucosal pustules (pyostomatitis vegetans) (Figure 4.169).

Diagnosis

- Biopsy;
- Full blood picture;
- Sigmoidoscopy and colonoscopy;
- Barium enema.

Management

- Systemic sulphasalazine or corticosteroids;
- Haematinics are needed to correct any secondary deficiencies;
- Topical corticosteroids may be helpful.

Varicella-zoster virus infections

See Chickenpox, Zoster

Verruciform xanthoma

Definition

A warty lesion which contains xanthoma cells

Incidence

Rare

Age mainly affected

Middle-aged and elderly

Sex mainly affected

M=F

Aetiology

Unknown. Probably a reactive lesion, it may be associated with:

- Naevi;
- Bone marrow transplantation;
- Graft-versus-host disease.

Clinical features

This is typically a solitary benign nodule which:

- May be asymptomatic;
- Is papular and firm;
- Is typically <1 cm diameter;
- May be white or, more commonly, yellowish or reddish;
- Is usually seen on the gingiva, alveolus or palate.

Diagnosis

- Biopsy;
- Blood biochemistry shows no hyperlipidaemia.

Management

Excise

Vitamin deficiencies

Deficiencies of haematinics such as vitamins B and folic acid, and iron, even in the pre-anaemic stage can give rise to:

- Angular stomatitis (Figure 4.179);

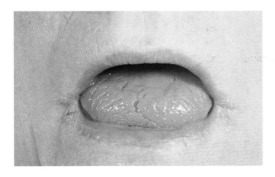

Figure 4.179
Angular stomatitis in an elderly vitamin-deficient and anaemic patient

- Glossitis;
- Ulcers;
- Sore mouth in the absence of obvious clinical lesions (burning mouth syndrome).

Vitamin C deficiency may cause scurvy (Chapter 6). The cause of the deficiency should be sought and rectified and the deficiency corrected. Oral lesions then typically resolve.

Warts

Incidence

Uncommon. A higher prevalence is seen in patients with sexually transmitted diseases or who are immunocompromised.

Age mainly affected

Verrucae are usually seen on the lips of children who have warts on the fingers. Condylomata are usually seen on the tongue or fauces in sexually active adults.

Sex mainly affected

M=F

Aetiology

Papillomaviruses: usually transmitted from:

- Skin lesions (verruca vulgaris); HPV 2, 4, 40 or 57;
- Occasionally from anogenital lesions (condyloma acuminata); HPV 6, 11, 16 or 18;
- In HIV disease, HPV 7, 72 or 73 may be found.

Clinical features

- Either can be warty papules or more smooth-surfaced;
- Verrucae are found predominantly on the lips;
- Condyloma acuminata are found on the tongue (Figure 4.180) or palate.

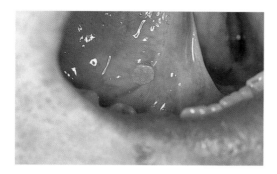

Figure 4.180
Wart; a genital wart
(condyloma acuminatum)

Diagnosis and management

Excision biopsy or cryosurgery, topical podophyllin 20% in tincture of benzoin, or intralesional alpha interferon. Imiquimod is a new antiviral under trial.

Wegener's granulomatosis (disseminated malignant granuloma)

Definition

This is a potentially lethal disseminating necrotizing granulomatous condition.

Incidence

Rare

Age mainly affected

Adults

Sex mainly affected

M=F

Aetiology

Unknown; though *Staphylococcus aureus* has been implicated.

Clinical features

This typically:

- Initially affects the respiratory tract;
- Is followed by widespread arteritis of small vessels, and renal damage (glomerulonephritis);
- May cause orofacial lesions including:
  - Persistent sinusitis;
  - Persistent oral ulceration, especially buccally or on tongue;
  - Non-healing extraction socket;
  - Painless, progressive gingival enlargement that may have a fairly characteristic 'strawberry-like' appearance. Swelling of the gingiva in a previously healthy mouth, particularly if associated with swollen, inflamed papillae, should arouse suspicion of this condition.
- May also produce:
  - Nasal obstruction;
  - Serous otitis media;
  - Weight loss;
  - Fever.

Diagnosis

- Lesional biopsy;
- Serology; antineutrophil cytoplasmic antibodies (ANCA);
- Chest radiography;
- Pulmonary and renal investigations.

Management

Cytotoxic therapy is usually needed, typically cyclophosphamide, though there are reports of beneficial responses to antibiotics.

White sponge naevus (familial white folded gingivostomatosis)

Definition

White sponge naevus is an inherited condition of stratified squamous epithelia which manifests with symptomless white oral lesions.

Incidence

Rare

Age mainly affected

From birth

Sex mainly affected

M=F

Aetiology

Autosomal dominant defect in epithelial maturation, due to mutations in keratins 4 or 13, with hyperparakeratosis, acanthosis, intracellular oedema and impaired desquamation.

Clinical features

Asymptomatic, diffuse, bilateral white lesions with a shaggy or spongy, wrinkled surface (Figure 4.181) are seen:

- Typically on the buccal mucosa;
- Sometimes on the tongue, floor of mouth or elsewhere;
- Occasionally also in the pharynx, oesophagus, nose, genitals and anus (then sometimes called Cannon's disease);

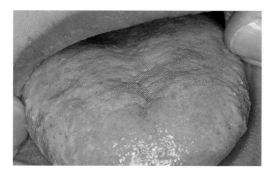

Figure 4.181
White sponge naevus

- The conjunctivae are not affected (c.f. benign intraepithelial dyskeratosis).

Diagnosis

Diagnosed from the clinical features, biopsy is confirmatory but rarely indicated. Differentiate from other congenital white lesions such as:

- Leukoedema;
- Pachyonychia congenita;
- Focal palmoplantar and oral mucosa hyperkeratosis syndrome;
- Dyskeratosis congenita;
- Benign intraepithelial dyskeratosis.

Management

No treatment is available or needed, other than reassurance.

Zoster (shingles)

Definition

Zoster is a painful unilateral rash in a dermatome due to reactivation of varicella-zoster virus (VZV) latent in the sensory ganglion of the dermatome.

Incidence

Uncommon

Age mainly affected

Elderly or immunocompromised patients, though rarely children may suffer if their mother had varicella during pregnancy.

Sex mainly affected

M=F

Aetiology

After primary infection, VZV remains latent in dorsal root ganglia, including the trigeminal ganglion in some patients. Reactivation of the VZV may result in herpes zoster.

Clinical features

Zoster, or shingles, is usually seen in elderly or immunocompromised persons such as AIDS patients. The thoracic region is mainly affected, but in 30% of sufferers, lesions are in the trigeminal region. Features include the following:

- Pain, which is unilateral, severe, and occurs before, during and sometimes after rash (postherpetic neuralgia);
- Rash, which is ipsilateral and in the distribution of the sensory nerve involved (dermatome), in a band-like pattern (hence zoster, Latin for belt). Like chickenpox, it goes through macular, papular, vesicular and pustular stages before crusting and healing, sometimes with scars;
- Mouth ulcers if the maxillary or mandibular divisions of the trigeminal nerve are involved:
  - Maxillary nerve involved—rash over ipsilateral cheek: ulcers and pain in ipsilateral plate and maxillary teeth (Figures 4.182 and 4.183);
  - Mandibular nerve involved—rash and pain over lower ipsilateral face and lip: ulcers and pain in tongue and soft tissues (Figures 4.184 and 4.185): pain also in mandibular teeth.

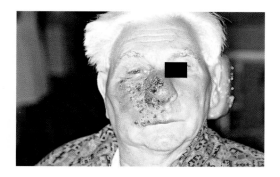

Figure 4.182
Zoster (shingles) of the maxillary division of the trigeminal nerve

Diagnosis

The diagnosis is usually clinically obvious, although, if the patient is seen before the rash appears, a misdiagnosis of toothache may be made.

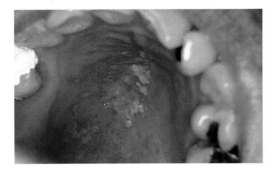

Figure 4.183
Maxillary zoster (shingles)

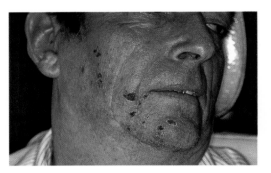

Figure 4.184
Mandibular zoster (shingles)

Figure 4.185
Mandibular zoster (shingles)

Management

- Exclude malignancy/immune defect (including HIV);
- Systemic aciclovir (high dose) orally or parenterally. This helps resolve zoster and reduces the incidence of postherpetic neuralgia, especially in immunocompromised patients (Table 15.9);
- Valaciclovir or famciclovir may be needed for aciclovir-resistant VZV infections (Table 10.9);
- Analgesics (Table 10.3);
- Anticonvulsants such as carbamazepine or sodium valproate may be needed to control neuralgia;
- Symptomatically treat mouth ulcers (Tables 10.1 and 10.2);
- If there is ophthalmic zoster obtain an urgent ophthalmological opinion since sight may be endangered.

Further reading

Almeida O, Scully C. Oral lesions in the systemic mycoses. *Curr Opin Dent* (1991) **1**: 423–8.

Axell T, Holmstrup P, Kramer IRH et al. International seminar on oral leuko-plakia and associated lesions related to tobacco habits. *Community Dent Oral Epidemiol* (1984) **12**: 145–54.

Barnard NA, Scully C, Eveson JW et al. Oral cancer development in patients with oral lichen planus. *Oral Pathol Med* (1993) **22**: 421–4.

Boyle P, MacFarlane GJ, Zheng T et al. Recent advances in the epidemiol-ogy of head and neck cancer. *Curr Opin Oncol* (1992) **4**: 471–7.

Boyle P, MacFarlane G, Scully C. Oral cancer: necessity for prevention strate-gies. *Lancet* (1993) **342**: 1129.

Burton J, Scully C. The lips. In: Champion RH, Burton J, Burns DA, Breathnach SM, eds, *Textbook of Dermatology*, 6th edn (Blackwells: Oxford, 1998).

Camisa C, Helm TN. Paraneoplastic pemphigus is a distinct neoplasia-induced autoimmune disease. *Arch Dermatol* (1993) **75**: 209–13.

Chorzelski TP, Jablonska S, Maciejowska E. Linear IgA bullous dermatosis of adults. *Clin Dermatol* (1991) **9**: 383–92.

Daley TD. Common acanthotic and keratotic lesions of the oral mucosa: a review. *J Can Dent Assoc* (1990) **56**: 407–9.

Dimitrakopoulos I, Zopuloumis L, Lazaridis N et al. Primary tuberculosis of the oral cavity. *Oral Surg Oral Med Oral Pathol* (1991) **72**: 712–15.

Epstein JB, Scully C. Herpes simplex virus in immunocompromised patients: growing evidence of drug resistance. *Oral Surg Oral Med Oral Pathol* (1991) **72**: 47–50.

Epstein J, Scully C. Neoplastic disease in the head and neck of patients with AIDS. *Int J Oral Maxillofac Surg* (1992) **2**: 219–26.

Epstein JB, Scully C. Cytomegalovirus: a virus of increasing relevance to oral medicine and pathology. *J Oral Pathol Med* (1993) **22**: 348–53.

Epstein JB, Scully C. Oral adverse effects of medical management in patients with HIV infection. *AIDS Patient Care* (1993) **Dec**: 304–11.

Epstein JB, Scully C. Assessing the patient at risk for oral squamous cell carcinoma. *Spec Care Dentist* (1997) **17**: 120–8.

Eversole LR. Immunopathology of oral mucosal ulcerative, desquamative and bullous diseases. Selective review of the literature. *Oral Surg Oral Med Oral Pathol* (1994) **77**: 555–71.

Eveson JW, Scully C. *Colour Atlas of Oral Pathology* (Mosby-Wolfe: London, 1995).

Firestein GS, Gruber HE, Weisman MH. Mouth and genital ulcers with inflamed cartilage: MAGIC syndrome. *Am J Med* (1985) **79**: 65–72.

Garlick JA, Taichman LB. Human papillomavirus infection of the oral mucosa. *Am J Dermatopathol* (1991) **13**: 386–95.

Gill Y, Scully C. Orofacial odontogenic infections: review of microbiology and current treatment. *Oral Surg Oral Med Oral Pathol* (1990) **70**: 155–8.

James J, Ferguson MM, Forsyth A et al. Oral lichenoid reactions related to mercury sensitivity. *Br J Oral Maxillofac Surg* (1987) **25**: 474–80.

Jarrett M. Herpes simplex infections. *Arch Dermatol* (1983) **119**: 99–103.

Jones JH, Mason DK. *Oral Manifestations of Systemic Disease*, 2nd edn (Baillière: London, 1980).

Jorizzo JL. Behçet's syndrome. *Arch Dermatol* (1986) **122**: 556–8.

Kaban LB, Mulliken JB. Vascular anomalies of the maxillofacial region. *J Oral Maxillofac Surg* (1986) **44**: 203–13.

Kano Y, Shiohara T, Yagita A et al. Association between cheilitis granulomatosa and Crohn's disease. *J Am Acad Dermatol* (1993) **28**: 801–2.

Kirtschig G, Wojnarowska F. Autoimmune blistering diseases: an update of diagnostic methods and investigations. *Clin Exp Dermatol* (1994) **19**: 97–112.

Lamey P-J, Carmichael F, Scully C. Oral pigmentation, Addison's disease and the results of screening for adreno-cortical insufficiency. *Br Dent J* (1985) **158**: 297–8.

Lamey P-J, Rees TD, Binnie WH et al. Oral presentation of pemphigus vulgaris and its response to systemic steroid therapy. *Oral Surg Oral Med Oral Pathol* (1992) **74**: 54–7.

Langdon J, Henk JM, eds, *Malignant Tumours of the Mouth, Jaws and Salivary Glands*, 2nd edn (Edward Arnold: London, 1995).

Laskaris GC, Sklavounov A, Stratigos J. Bullous pemphigoid, cicatricial pemphigoid and pemphigus vulgaris: a comparative clinical survey of 278 cases. *Oral Surg Oral Med Oral Pathol* (1982) **54**: 656–62.

Lozada-Nur F, Gorsky M, Silverman S. Oral erythema multiforme: clinical observations and treatment of 95 patients. *Oral Surg Oral Med Oral Pathol* (1989) **67**: 36–40.

McDonald JS, Crissman JD, Gluckman JL. Verrucous carcinoma of the oral cavity. *Head Neck Surg* (1982) **5**: 22–8.

Manton SM, Scully C. Mucous membrane pemphigoid: an elusive diagnosis. *Oral Surg Oral Med Oral Pathol* (1988) **66**: 37–40.

Manton SL, Eggleston SI, Alexander I et al. Oral presentation of secondary syphilis. *Br Dent J* (1986) **160**: 237–8.

Millard HD, Mason DK, eds, *Perspectives on 1993 World Workshop on Oral Medicine*. Ann Arbor: University of Michigan, 1995).

Miller CS, Redding SW. Diagnosis and management of orofacial herpes simplex virus infections. *Dent Clin North Am* (1992) **36**: 879–95.

Moyer GN, Terzhalmy GT, O'Brian JT. Nelson's syndrome: another condition associated with mucocutaneous hyperpigmentation. *J Oral Med* (1985) **1**: 13–17.

Nesbit SP, Gobetti JP. Multiple occurrences of oral erythema multiforme after secondary herpes simplex: report of a case and review of the literature. *J Am Dent Assoc* (1986) **112**: 348–52.

Neville B, Laden SA, Smith SE et al. Pyostomatitis vegetans. *Am J Dermatopathol* (1985) **7**: 69–77.

Odds FC. Candida infections: an overview. *CRC Crit Rev Microbiol* (1987) **15**: 1–5.

Pindborg JJ, Scully C. Orofacial manifestations of HIV infection. *Med Int* (1990) **76**: 3172–4.

Porter SR, Scully C. Aphthous stomatitis: an overview of aetiopathogenesis and management. *Clin Exp Dermatol* (1991) **16**: 235–43.

Porter SR, Scully C. HIV: the surgeon's perspective. 1: Update of pathogenesis, epidemiology, management and risk of nosocomial transmission. *Br J Oral Maxillofac Surg* (1994) **32**: 222–30.

Porter SR, Scully C. HIV: the surgeon's perspective. 2: Diagnosis and management of non-malignant oral manifestations. *Br J Oral Maxillofac Surg* (1994) **32**: 231–40.

Porter SR, Scully C. HIV: the surgeon's perspective. 3: Diagnosis and management of malignant neoplasms. *Br J Oral Maxillofac Surg* (1994) **32**: 241–7.

Porter SR, Scully C, eds, *Oral Healthcare for those with HIV and Other Special Needs.* (Science Reviews: Northwood, 1995).

Porter SR, Scully C, Luker J, Glover S. Oral manifestations of HIV infection. *Update* (1990) **40**: 1173–80.

Porter SR, Bain SE, Scully C. Linear IgA disease manifesting as recalcitrant desquamative gingivitis. *Oral Surg Oral Med Oral Pathol* (1992) **74**: 179–82.

Porter S, Haria S, Scully C et al. Chronic candidiasis, enamel hypoplasia and pigmentary anomalies. *Oral Surg Oral Med Oral Pathol* (1992) **73**: 312–14.

Porter SR, Scully C, Mutlu S. Viral infections affecting periodontal health. *Periodontal Clinical Investigations* (1995) **15**: 17–24.

Porter SR, Scully C, Pedersen A. Recurrent aphthous stomatitis. *Crit Rev Oral Biol Med* (1998) **9**: 306–21.

Samaranayake LP, Scully C. Oral disease and sexual medicine. *Br J Sexual Med* (1988) **15**: 138–43, 174–80.

Schiodt M. Oral manifestations of lupus erythematosus. *Oral Surg Oral Med Oral Pathol* (1984) **13**: 101–47.

Scully C. Orofacial herpes simplex virus infections: current concepts on the epidemiology, pathogenesis and treatment and disorders in which the virus may be implicated. *Oral Surg Oral Med Oral Pathol* (1989) **68**: 701–10.

Scully C. Treatment of oral lichen planus (leading article). *Lancet* (1990) **336**: 913–14.

Scully C. Oral manifestations of HIV: less common lesions. *Dermatol Digest* (1991) **6**: 20–2.

Scully C. Oral manifestations of HIV: more common lesions. *Dermatol Digest* (1991) **5**: 27–8.

Scully C. Oral infections in the immunocompromised patient. *Br Dent J* (1992) **172**: 401–7.

Scully C. Are viruses associated with aphthae and oral vesiculobullous disorders. *Br J Oral Maxillofac Surg* (1993) **31**: 173–7.

Scully C. Clinical diagnostic methods for the detection of premalignant and early malignant oral lesions. *Community Dent Health* (1993) **1** (Supplement 1): 43–52.

Scully C. Diagnosis and diagnostic procedures: general and soft tissue diagnosis. In: *Pathways in Practice.* (Faculty of General Dental Practice, Royal College of Surgeons of England: London, 1993) 25–33.

Scully C. Inflammatory disorders of the oral mucosa. In: English GM, ed., *Otolaryngology.* (Lippincott: Philadelphia, 1993) 1–28.

Scully C. Oral cancer: new insights into pathogenesis. *Dent Update* (1993) **20**: 95–100.

Scully C. The pathology of orofacial disease. In: Barnes IE, Walls AWG, eds, *Gerodontology.* (Wright-Butterworths: Oxford, 1994) 29–41.

Scully C. Oral precancer: preventive and medical approaches to management. *Oral Oncology* (1995) **31**: 16–26.

Scully C. Prevention of oral mucosal disease. In: Murray JJ, ed., *Prevention of Oral and Dental Disease*, 3rd edn. (Oxford University Press: Oxford, 1995) 160–72.

Scully C. New aspects of oral viral diseases. *Curr Top Pathol* (1996) **90**: 30–96

Scully C. The oral cavity. In: Champion RH, Burton J, Ebling FJG, eds, *Textbook of Dermatology*, 6th edn (Blackwells: Oxford, 1998).

Scully C, Almeida O. Orofacial manifestations of the systemic mycoses. *J Oral Pathol Oral Med* (1992) **21**: 289–94.

Scully C, Bagg J. Viral infections in dentistry. *Curr Opin Dent* (1992) **9**: 8–11.

Scully C, Cawson RA. Potentially malignant oral lesions. *J Epidemiol Biostat* (1996) **1**: 3–12.

Scully C, Cawson RA. *Medical Problems in Dentistry*, 4th edn. (Butterworth-Heinemann: Oxford, 1998).

Scully C, Epstein JB. Oral health care for the cancer patient. *Eur J Cancer B Oral Oncol* (1996) **32**: 281–92.

Scully C, Eveson JW. Oral granulomatosis (leading article). *Lancet* (1991) **338**: 20–1.

Scully C, McCarthy G. Management of oral health in persons with HIV infection. *Oral Surg Oral Med Oral Pathol* (1992) **73**: 215–25.

Scully C, Porter SR. Diseases of the oral mucosa. *Med Int* (1990) **76**: 3154–62.

Scully C, Porter SR. An ABC of oral health care in patients with HIV infection. *Br Dent J* (1991) **170**: 149–50.

Scully C, Porter SR. Oral medicine: 2. Disorders affecting the oral mucosa (part 1). *Postgrad Dent* (1992) **2**: 109–13.

Scully C, Porter SR. Oral mucosal disease: a decade of new entities, aetiologies and associations. *Int Dent J* (1994) **44**: 33–43.

Scully C. Management of the sore mouth: other causes of oral soreness. *Eur J Palliat Care* (1995) **2** (Supplement 1): 13–15.

Scully C, Ward-Booth P. Detection and treatment of early cancers of the oral cavity. *Crit Rev Oncol/Haematol* (1995) **21**: 63–75.

Scully C, Welbury R. *Colour Atlas of Oral Disease in Children and Adolescents*. (Mosby-Wolfe: London, 1994).

Scully C, Midda M, Eveson JW. Adult linear immunoglobulin. A disease manifesting as desquamative gingivitis. *Oral Surg Oral Med Oral Pathol* (1990) **70**: 45–3.

Scully C, Epstein JB, Porter S, Luker J. Recognition of oral lesions of HIV infection 2. Hairy leukoplakia and Kaposi's sarcoma. *Br Dent J* (1990) **169**: 332–3.

Scully C, Epstein JB, Porter S, Luker J. Recognition of oral lesions of HIV infection. 3. Gingival and periodontal disease and less common lesions. *Br Dent J* (1990) **169**: 370–2.

Scully C, Epstein JB, Porter SR, Luker J. Recognition of oral lesions of HIV infection. 1. Candidosis. *Br Dent J* (1990) **169**: 295–6.

Scully C, Epstein JB, Porter SR, Cox M. Viruses and chronic diseases involving the human oral mucosa. *Oral Surg Oral Med Oral Pathol* (1991) **72**: 537–44.

Scully C, Epstein J, Porter S et al. Viruses and chronic disorders involving the human oral mucosa. *Oral Surg Oral Med Oral Pathol* (1991) **72**: 537–44.

Scully C, Laskaris G, Pindborg J, Porter SR, Reichart P. Oral manifestations of HIV infection and their management. 1. More common lesions. *Oral Surg Oral Med Oral Pathol* (1991) **71**: 158–66.

Scully C, Laskaris G, Pindborg J et al. Oral manifestations of HIV infection and their management. 2. Less common lesions. *Oral Surg Oral Med Oral Pathol* (1991) **71**: 167–71.

Scully C, Boyle P, Tedesco B. The recognition and diagnosis of cancer arising in the mouth. *Postgrad Doctor* (1992) **15**: 134–41 and *Postgrad Dent* (1995) **5**: 42–7.

Scully C, El-Kabir M, Samaranayake LP. Candida and oral candidosis. *Crit Rev Oral Biol Med* (1994) **5**: 124–58.

Scully C, Almeida OPD, Warnakulasuriya KAAS, Johnson NW. Orofacial involvement by systemic mycoses in HIV infection. *Oral Dis* (1995) **1**: 61–2.

Scully C, Flint S, Porter S. *Oral Diseases.* (Martin Dunitz: London, 1996).

Scully C, Almeida ODP, Sposto MR. Deep mycoses in HIV infection. *Oral Dis* (1997) **3** (Supplement 1) 200–7.

Scully C, Beyli M, Feirrero M et al. Update on oral lichen planus: aetiopatho-genesis and management. *Crit Rev Oral Biol Med* (1998) **9**: 86–122.

Shklar G. Oral leukoplakia. *N Engl J Med* (1986) **315**: 1544–5.

Sigurgeirsson B, Lindelof B. Lichen planus and malignancy. An epidemio-logic study of 2071 patients and a review of the literature. *Arch Dermatol* (1991) **127**: 1684–8.

Silverman S, Gorsky M, Lozada-Nur F et al. Oral mucous membrane pem-phigoid. *Oral Surg Oral Med Oral Pathol* (1986) **61**: 233–7.

Singh N, Scully C, Joynston-Bechal S. Oral complications of cancer therapies: prevention and management. *Clin Oncol* (1996) **8**: 15–24.

Spruance SL. The natural history of recurrent oral-facial herpes simplex virus infection. *Semin Dermatol* (1992) **11**: 200–6.

Stal S, Hamilton S, Spira M. Haemangioma, lymphangioma and vascular malfor-mations of the head and neck. *Otolaryngol Clin North Am* (1986) **19**: 769–96.

Stephenson P, Lamey P-J, Scully C et al. Angina bullosa haemorrhagica: clin-ical and laboratory features in 30 patients. *Oral Surg Oral Med Oral Pathol* (1987) **63**: 560–5.

Stephenson P, Scully C, Prime SS et al. Angina bullosa haemorrhagica: lesional immunostaining and haematological findings. *Br J Oral Maxillofac Surg* (1987) **25**: 488–91.

Thomas I, Janniger CK. Hand, foot and mouth disease. *Cutis* (1993) **52**: 265–6.

Thornhill MH, Zakrzewska JM, Gilkes JJH. Pyostomatitis vegetans: report of three cases and review of the literature. *J Oral Pathol Med* (1992) **21**: 128–33.

Tradati N, Grigolat R, Calabrese L et al. Oral leukoplakias; to treat or not? *Oral Oncol* (1997) **33**: 317–22.

Triantos D, Porter SR, Scully C, Teo CG. Oral hairy leukoplakia; clinico-pathological features, pathogenesis, diagnosis and clinical significance. *Clin Infect Dis* (1997) **25**: 1392–6.

Vincent SD, Lilly GE. Clinical, historic and therapeutic features of aphthous stomatitis. Literature review and open clinical trial employing steroids. *Oral Surg Oral Med Oral Pathol* (1992) **74**: 79–86.

Vincent SD, Lilly GE, Baker KA. Clinical, historic and therapeutic features of cicatricial pemphigoid. *Oral Surg Oral Med Oral Pathol* (1993) **76**: 453–9.

van der Waal RI, Snow GB, Karim AB et al. Primary malignancy melanoma of the oral cavity: a review of eight cases. *Br Dent J* (1994) **176**: 185–8.

Ward-Booth P, Scully C. The management of mouth cancer. *Postgrad Doctor* (1992) **15**: 166–175 and *Postgrad Dent* (1995) **5**: 65–71.

Wechsler B, Piette JC. Behçet's disease. Retains most of its mysteries. *BMJ* (1992) **304**: 1199–200 (edit).

Wiesenfeld D, Martin A, Scully C et al. Oral manifestations in linear IgA disease. *Br Dent J* (1982) **153**: 389–99.

Weisenfeld DW, Ferguson MM, Mitchell D et al. Orofacial granulomatosis: a clinical and pathological analysis. *Q J Med* (1985) **54**: 101–13.

Winnie R, DeLuke DM. Melkersson–Rosenthal syndrome. *Int J Oral Maxillofac Surg* (1992) **21**: 115–17.

Yancey KM. The diagnosis and biology of bullous diseases. *Arch Dermatol* (1994) **130**: 983–7.

Zimmer WM, Rogers RS, Reeve CM et al. Orofacial manifestations of Melkersson–Rosenthal syndrome. *Oral Surg Oral Med Oral Pathol* (1992) **74**: 610–19.

5

Salivary disorders

Saliva is essential to oral health: patients who lack salivary flow suffer from lack of oral lubrication, and may develop infections as a consequence of the reduced defences. There is a range of causes of a reduction in salivary flow but drugs are the most common cause (Chapter 1). Causes of salivary gland swelling include inflammatory lesions (mumps, ascending sialadenitis, recurrent parotitis, HIV parotitis, Sjögren's syndrome, sarcoidosis), neoplasms, duct obstruction or sialosis.

Adenomatoid hyperplasia

See Chapter 8, page 344

Duct obstruction

Definition

Obstruction to a salivary duct is usually due to an internal blockage from a stone (calculus), mainly seen in the submandibular duct.

Incidence

Uncommon

Age mainly affected

Adults

Sex mainly affected

M=F

Aetiology

Calculi caused by stasis, strictures, mucus plugs or neoplasms are causes. Rarely, patients present with 'physiological' duct obstruction due either to duct spasm or an abnormal passage of the parotid duct through the buccinator or in relation to the masseter muscles.

Clinical features

Features include:

- Salivary gland swelling: unilateral, painful and intermittent, appearing just before, or at mealtimes (Figures 5.1 and 5.19). In older patients, this history is not always obtained; there may just be dull pain over the affected gland, referred elsewhere;
- Lack of swelling at other times.

Prolonged duct obstruction produces atrophy, particularly of serous acini.

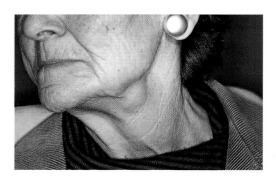

Figure 5.1
Submandibular salivary swelling from obstruction by calculus

Diagnosis

- It is possible clinically to determine the cause of major duct obstruction when a calculus is palpable or visible (Figures 5.2 and 5.20);

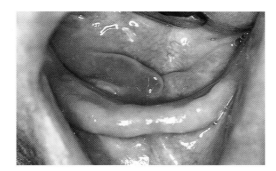

Figure 5.2
Sialolithiasis in the right submandibular duct

- Plain radiographs may reveal a calculus but nearly 50% are radio-lucent;
- Sialography should help differentiate the various causes of major duct obstruction. Extraductal causes of obstruction may be evident only on combined sialography and computerized tomography.

Management

Obstructions are overcome by surgical removal of the obstruction (such as a calculus), lithotripsy or duct dilatation.

Mucocele (mucous retention cyst; mucous cyst; ranula; myxoid cyst)

Definition

A cystic space filled with mucinous material

Incidence

Common

Age mainly affected

From childhood

Sex mainly affected

M>F

Aetiology

Usually there is rupture of the duct of a minor salivary gland consequent on minor trauma. Occasionally a mucocele results from retention of saliva because of duct obstruction.

Clinical features

Mucoceles appear as dome-shaped, translucent whitish-blue cystic lesions, papules or nodules. There are three main types:

*   Extravasation mucoceles due to mucus extravasating into the lamina propria. These are seen most commonly, especially in the lower lip to one side of the midline (Figures 5.3 and 5.4);
*   Mucoceles of the retention type; those in the floor of the mouth may resemble a frog's belly and are known therefore as ranulae (Figure 5.5). These are unilateral;
*   Superficial mucoceles due to extravasation of mucus beneath the epithelium which may mimic a vesiculobullous disorder.

Diagnosis

Care should be taken to ensure that the lesion is not a salivary gland tumour with cystic change, especially when dealing with an apparent mucous cyst in the *upper* lip.

Management

*   Superficial mucoceles usually resolve spontaneously;
*   The other mucoceles can be excised but they also respond well to cryosurgery, using a single freeze–thaw cycle.

Mumps (acute viral sialadenitis parotitis)

Definition

An acute infectious disease which principally affects the parotid salivary glands

Incidence

Common

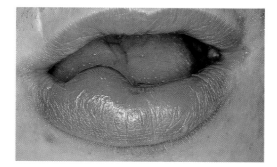

Figure 5.3
Mucocele in typical site

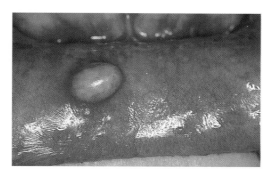

Figure 5.4
Mucocele in typical site

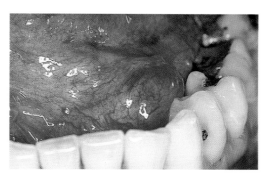

Figure 5.5
Mucocele in floor of mouth

Age mainly affected

Children

Sex mainly affected

M=F

Aetiology

Usually infection with an RNA paramyxovirus, the mumps virus. Rarely Coxsackie, ECHO, EBV, CMV, HCV or HIV infection

Clinical features

Transmission of classical mumps is by direct contact or by droplet spread from saliva. An incubation period of 2–3 weeks elapses before clinical features appear.

- Parotitis: acute onset of painful, usually bilaterally, enlarged parotids (Figure 5.6), although in the early stages only one parotid gland may appear to be involved. The submandibular glands may also be affected;
- The skin over the affected glands appears normal, as does the saliva; features which help distinguish from acute bacterial siladenitis;
- Trismus;
- Fever and malaise.

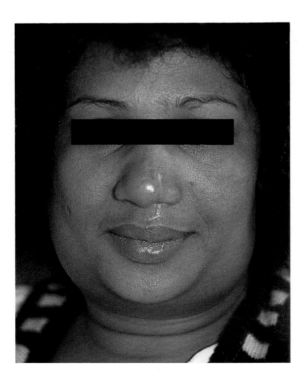

Figure 5.6
Mumps

Extrasalivary manifestations may include:

- Inflammation of the testes (orchitis) or ovaries (oophoritis). Ensuing infertility is rare;
- Pancreatitis;
- Meningitis or meningoencephalitis;
- Deafness.

Diagnosis

The diagnosis is clinical, but confirmation, if needed, is by demonstrating:

- A four-fold rise in serum antibody titres between acute serum and convalescent serum taken 3 weeks later;
- Raised levels of serum amylases or lipases.

Management

- No specific antiviral agents are available;
- Treatment is symptomatic, involving analgesics, adequate hydration and reducing the fever.

Patient isolation for 6–10 days may be advised since the virus is in saliva during this time. Prevention is by immunization, now carried out in childhood.

Necrotizing sialometaplasia

Definition

Benign self-limiting inflammatory salivary disorder

Incidence

Rare

Age mainly affected

Adults, 5th decade

Sex mainly affected

M>F

Aetiology

Unknown but it appears to result from infarction and is seen especially in smokers.

Clinical features

This is typically:

- Initially an asymptomatic swelling;
- Of sudden onset;
- In the palate, though any oral tissue may be affected;
- Followed by painful solitary ulceration (Figure 5.7);
- Self-limiting, healing over 5 to 8 weeks.

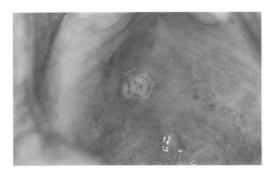

Figure 5.7
*Necrotizing
sialometaplasia*

Diagnosis

- Clinical features;
- Biopsy (may show pseudo epitheliomatous hyperplasia).

Management

This is a self-limiting condition but may take 1–2 months to heal completely.

Recurrent parotitis of childhood

Definition

Repeated unilateral parotitis and sialectasis in a child or adolescent

Incidence

Uncommon

Age mainly affected

Children

Sex mainly affected

M>F

Aetiology

Most cases appear related to congenital duct anomalies; sialectasis is demonstrable by sialography.

Clinical features

Intermittent, unilateral parotid swelling which lasts 2–3 weeks with spontaneous regression. It may occur simultaneously or alternately on the contralateral side. There is little pain.

Diagnosis

This is a clinical diagnosis.

Management

No specific treatment is available or required. Repeated courses of antimicrobials are often used but usually the condition resolves after puberty.

Salivary neoplasms

Benign neoplasms include:

- Pleomorphic adenoma;
- Monomorphic adenoma;
- Papillary cystadenoma lymphomatosum.

Malignant neoplasms include:

- Mucoepidermoid carcinoma;
- Adenoid cystic carcinoma;
- Acinic cell carcinoma;
- Polymorphous low-grade carcinoma.

Incidence

Uncommon

Age mainly affected

Older adults

Sex mainly affected

F>M

Aetiology

The aetiology of salivary neoplasms is unclear. Viruses may be involved; polyoma viruses have been implicated in animal models, and other viruses, such as EBV in some human neoplasms. Irradiation has been implicated in some tumours.

Clinical features

A wide range of different neoplasms can affect the salivary glands. **Tumours of the major salivary glands** mostly:

- Present as unilateral swelling of the parotid (Figure 5.8);
- Are benign;
- Are pleomorphic adenomas; the next most common tumour is carcinoma which, in some cases, arises in a long-standing pleomorphic salivary adenoma.

The 'rule of nines' is an approximation that states that nine out of 10 tumours affect the parotid, nine out of 10 are benign and nine out of 10 are pleomorphic salivary adenomas (PSAs). **Intraoral salivary gland neoplasms** are:

- Less common than in major glands;
- Malignant in a higher proportion;

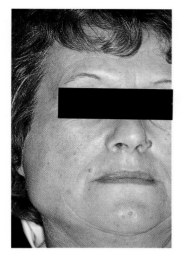

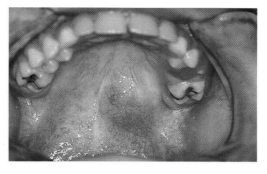

Figure 5.9
Palatal pleomorphic adenoma

Figure 5.8
*Parotid pleomorphic
adenoma*

- Typically unilateral;
- Mainly pleomorphic adenoma, but adenoid cystic carcinoma and mucoepidermoid carcinoma are relatively more common in the mouth than in the major glands;
- Most common in the palate (Figure 5.9) but may be seen in the buccal mucosa or upper lip; rarely in the tongue or lower lip.

Most tumours in the:

- Parotid gland are PSAs and benign;
- Submandibular gland are PSAs and benign but one-third are malignant;
- Sublingual gland are malignant;
- Tongue are malignant, especially adenoid cystic carcinoma;
- Lips are benign (pleomorphic or other adenoma), and seen in the upper lip.

Classification

The World Health Organization classification is the most widely used (Table 5.1), and the epithelial tumours, which are the most important, can be memorized by the mnemonic: *A Most Acceptable Classification.*

Table 5.1 Classification of salivary gland epithelial tumours (after World Health Organization)

Adenomas*
  Pleomorphic
  Monomorphic
    Adenolymphoma
    Oxyphilic
    Others
Mucoepidermoid†
Acinic cell tumours†
Carcinomas‡
  Adenoid cystic
  Adenocarcinoma
  Epidermoid
  Polymorphous low-grade adenocarcinoma
  Undifferentiated carcinoma in pleomorphic adenoma

*Benign; †intermediate; ‡malignant.

Adenomas

The **pleomorphic salivary adenoma** (PSA; mixed salivary gland tumour) is:

- The most common salivary gland neoplasm;
- Usually slow growing (Figure 5.10);
- A lobulated, rubbery swelling with normal overlying skin or mucosa but a bluish appearance if intraoral (Figures 5.11–5.13);
- Usually benign;
- Poorly encapsulated and in intimate relationship with the facial nerve.

Malignant change is rare but is suggested clinically by:

- Rapid growth;
- Pain;
- Fixation to deep tissues;
- Facial palsy.

Unlike the pleomorphic adenoma, **monomorphic adenomas** have a uniform cellular structure of epithelial elements. They include:

- **Adenolymphoma** (Papillary cystadenoma lymphomatosum or Warthin's tumour), found only in the parotid and benign;

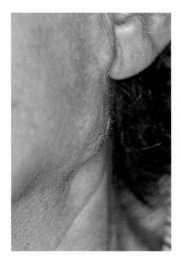

Figure 5.10
Pleomorphic adenoma in the parotid

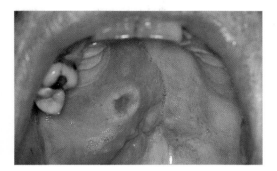

Figure 5.11
Pleomorphic adenoma

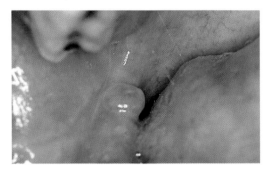

Figure 5.12
Pleomorphic adenoma

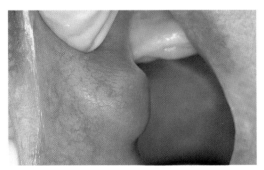

Figure 5.13
Pleomorphic adenoma

- **Oxyphil adenoma**: this rare neoplasm is found virtually only in the parotid, affects mainly the elderly and is benign.

Mucoepidermoid tumours are usually slow-growing, of low-grade malignancy.

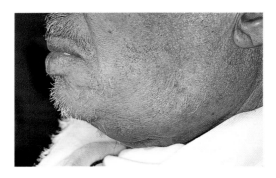

Figure 5.14
Adenoid cystic carcinoma (cylindroma) in the submandibular gland

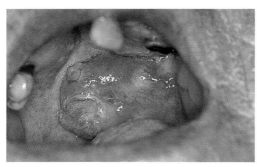

Figure 5.15
Adenoid cystic carcinoma

Acinic cell tumours are very rare and, though all grades of malignancy have been reported, are often benign.

Most **carcinomas** metastasize late. Some tumours, such as adenoid cystic carcinoma, invade bone and neural tissues preferentially.

- **Adenoid cystic carcinoma** (cylindroma) is slow-growing, malignant (Figures 5.14 and 5.15) and infiltrates perineurally and metastasizes;
- **Adenocarcinoma** is rapidly growing and more malignant than adenoid cystic carcinoma;
- **Epidermoid carcinoma** is often undifferentiated and highly malignant;
- **Polymorphous low-grade adenocarcinoma** is slow-growing, seen mainly in minor glands in older females, and rarely metastasizes.

Diagnosis

Early detection carries a good prognosis.

- A swelling of a salivary gland, especially if localized, firm and persistent, may be a neoplasm. A long history of gradual gland enlargement suggests a benign process, while pain or facial nerve palsy is ominous and suggests carcinoma (see above);

- Some tumours may be small and the presentation may be of pain only;
- Sialography may reveal an obvious filling defect or displacement of the gland but is a relatively imprecise means of tumour detection;
- Computerized tomography (CT) is a more sensitive means of tumour detection;
- Ultrasonography has a limited application;
- Biopsy. Preoperative needle biopsy, sometimes CT guided, has a high tumour detection rate in experienced hands. The diagnosis can often best be firmly established by open biopsy, but this is best carried out at the time of definitive operation, in order to avoid seeding malignant cells.

Management

- Surgical excision;
- Radiotherapy is sometimes an adjunct.

Sialadenitis; acute bacterial ascending

Definition

Sialadenitis due to bacterial infection ascending from the oral cavity

Incidence

Rare

Age mainly affected

Older adults

Sex mainly affected

M=F

Aetiology

The parotid glands are most commonly affected by ascending sialadenitis, which may be seen:

- After radiotherapy to the head and neck;

- In Sjögren's syndrome;
- Occasionally following gastrointestinal surgery, because of dehydration and dry mouth;
- Rarely in otherwise apparently healthy patients, when it is usually due to salivary abnormalities such as calculi, mucus plugs and duct strictures.

The organisms most commonly isolated are *Streptococcus viridans* and *Staphylococcus aureus* (often penicillin-resistant).

Clinical features

Acute sialadenitis typically presents with:

- Painful and tender enlargement of one salivary gland only;
- The overlying skin possibly reddened (Figure 5.16);
- Pus exuding from, or milked from the salivary duct orifice (Figure 5.17);
- Trismus;
- Cervical lymphadenopathy;
- Pyrexia.

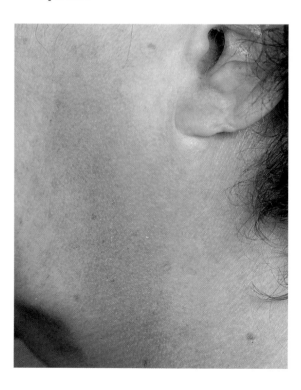

Figure 5.16
Acute bacterial sialadenitis

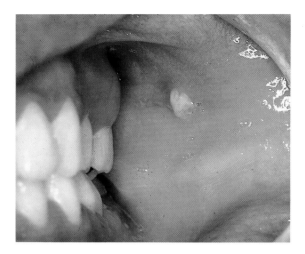

Figure 5.17
*Acute bacterial
sialadenitis; pus
from parotid duct*

If the infection localizes as a parotid abscess, it may point externally through the overlying skin or, rarely, into the external acoustic meatus.

Diagnosis

The diagnosis is essentially clinical, but pus should be sent for culture and sensitivity testing.

Management

- Prompt antimicrobial therapy. Amoxicillin 3 g then 250 mg three times daily for 5–7 days is indicated (flucloxacillin if *Staphylococcus* and not allergic to penicillin; erythromycin in penicillin allergy);
- Analgesia;
- Surgical drainage is needed where fluctuation is present, as there may be extensive glandular damage;
- Hydration must be ensured;
- Salivation should be stimulated by chewing gum or use of sialogogues.

Sialadenitis; chronic bacterial

Definition

Chronic infection of a salivary gland

Incidence

Rare

Age mainly affected

Older adults

Sex mainly affected

M=F

Aetiology

Chronic bacterial sialadenitis may develop after acute sialadenitis, particularly if inappropriate antibiotics are used or predisposing factors are not eliminated. Chronic sialadenitis may follow salivary calculus formation. Unfortunately, serous acini may atrophy when salivary outflow is chronically obstructed and this further reduces function.

Clinical features

- The affected salivary gland is chronically swollen;
- Gland often not tender;
- No systemic features of infection.

Diagnosis

Clinical and radiography

Management

Surgical excision is often needed but occasionally the duct is ligated.

Sialosis (sialadenosis)

Definition

Sialosis is bilaterally symmetrical painless enlargement of salivary glands.

Incidence

Uncommon

Age mainly affected

Adults

Sex mainly affected

M>F

Aetiology

Dysregulation of the autonomic innervation of the salivary glands is the unifying factor in a variety of causes recognized which include:

- **Alcoholism**: alcohol abuse with or without accompanying liver cirrhosis;
- **Endocrine conditions**: diabetes mellitus, acromegaly, thyroid disease, pregnancy;
- **Nutritional disorders**: anorexia nervosa, bulimia, cystic fibrosis with malnutrition;
- **Drugs**: sympathomimetic drugs such as isoprenaline.

Clinical features

These include:

- Salivary gland swelling; soft, painless and typically bilateral (usually the parotids) (Figure 5.18);
- No xerostomia;

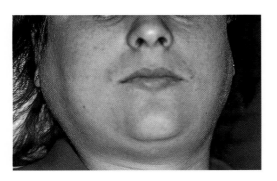

Figure 5.18
Sialosis

- No trismus;
- No fever.

Diagnosis

- The diagnosis of sialosis is one of exclusion, based mainly on history and clinical examination;
- Blood examination for antibodies indicative of Sjögren's syndrome (page 266), raised glucose levels, possibly growth hormone levels or abnormal liver function may point to an underlying cause;
- Salivary biopsy is not usually needed;
- Salivary gland function is normal;
- Sialography is likely to show enlarged normal glands;
- Sialochemistry may show raised potassium and calcium levels which would not be present in salivary enlargement due to other causes.

Management

No specific treatment is available but sialosis may resolve when alcohol intake is reduced or glucose control instituted.

Sialolithiasis

See page 245

Definition

Calculus, usually in a salivary duct

Incidence

Uncommon

Age mainly affected

Older adults

Sex mainly affected

M=F

Aetiology

Possibly salivary stasis

Clinical features

Salivary calculi (sialoliths):

- Usually affect the submandibular duct;
- May present with pain in, and swelling of, the gland; particularly around mealtimes (Figures 5.1 and 5.19);
- Are sometimes asymptomatic;
- Are usually yellow or white and can sometimes be seen in the duct (Figures 5.2 and 5.20);
- May be palpable;
- Are commonly radiopaque.

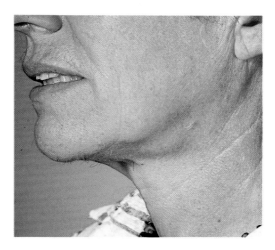

Figure 5.19
Sialolithiasis

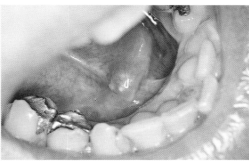

Figure 5.20
Sialolithiasis

Calculi are even less common in the parotid and then are typically radiolucent.

Diagnosis

Radiography; sialography if necessary

Management

Surgical or lithotripsy removal of obstruction

Sialorrhoea

See Chapter 1

Sjögren's syndrome

Definition

Sjögren's syndrome (SS) is the association of dry mouth (xerostomia) and dry eyes (keratoconjunctivitis sicca). *Primary* SS (SS-1 or sicca syndrome) is the term given when these features alone are present, but if a connective tissue disease or primary biliary cirrhosis is present, the term *secondary* SS (SS-2) is used. This is more common.

Incidence

Uncommon

Age mainly affected

Elderly

Sex mainly affected

F>M

Aetiology

An autoimmune inflammatory exocrinopathy which appears to be the result of lymphocyte-mediated destruction of salivary, lachrymal and

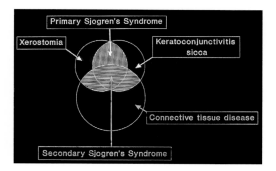

Figure 5.21
Sjögren's syndrome components

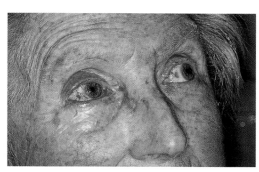

Figure 5.22
Eye soreness in Sjögren's syndrome

other exocrine glands (Figure 5.21). There may be a viral aetiology, possibly human retrovirus 5 (HRV-5), an endogenous retrovirus or HTLV-1, and a genetic predisposition. Hepatitis C virus and HIV can cause similar manifestations.

Clinical features

SS is a chronic multisystem disease which presents mainly with the following:

- Eye complaints include sensations of grittiness, soreness or dryness. The eyes may be red with infection of the conjunctivae and soft crusts at the angles (keratoconjunctivitis sicca: Figure 5.22). The lachrymal glands may swell;
- Other complaints; arthritis, dry vagina, purpura and many others;
- Oral complaints (often presenting features) include:
  - xerostomia;
  - difficulty eating dry foods such as biscuits (the cracker sign);
  - soreness;
  - difficulties in controlling dentures in speech and swallowing;
  - the salivary glands may swell;
  - unpleasant taste or loss of sense of taste (Chapter 1).

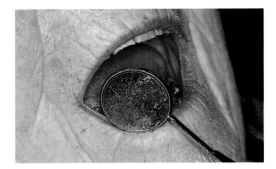

Figure 5.23
Dry mouth; debris on the examining dental mirror

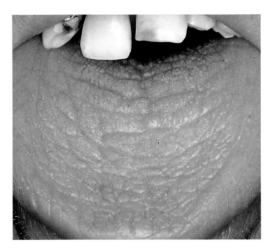

Figure 5.24
Dry mouth in Sjögren's syndrome

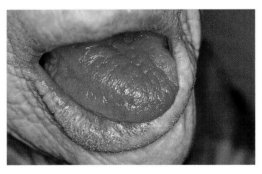

Figure 5.25
Dry mouth

The dryness of the mouth may be recognized by:

- The clicking quality of the speech as the tongue tends to stick to the palate;
- The mucosa tending to stick to a dental mirror (Figure 5.23);

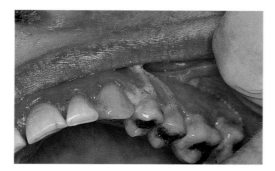

Figure 5.26
Dry mouth showing scant, frothy saliva

- The mouth may appear dry (Figure 5.24). In advanced cases the mucosa is obviously dry and glazed. The tongue typically also develops a characteristic lobulated, usually red, surface with partial or complete depapillation (Figure 5.25);
- There may be lack of the usual pooling of saliva in the floor of the mouth;
- Thin lines of frothy, viscous saliva along lines of contact of the oral soft tissues (Figure 5.26).

In SS-1, oral involvement may be more severe and recurrent sialadenitis, eye involvement and lymphoma may be more common.

Complications

- Soreness and redness of the oral mucosa, and angular stomatitis are usually the result of candidiasis, which is common;
- Dental caries tend to be severe and difficult to control, and may affect smooth surfaces and other areas not usually susceptible;
- Ascending (suppurative) sialadenitis is a hazard;
- Although mild enlargement of salivary glands is not uncommon in Sjögren's syndrome, it is occasionally massive and associated with enlargement of the regional lymph nodes, a condition called pseudolymphoma. The B-cell lymphoproliferation may actually become malignant, with a true lymphoma in some cases (Figure 5.27).

Diagnosis

The diagnosis of Sjögren's syndrome is mainly on:

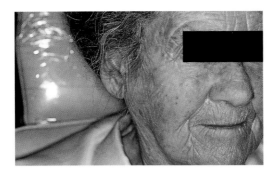

Figure 5.27
Lymphoma in right parotid gland complicating Sjögren's syndrome

- The history;
- Clinical examination;
- Autoantibodies—particularly antinuclear factor and rheumatoid factor and antinuclear antibodies known as SS-A (Ro) and SS-B (La);
- Anaemia;
- Raised erythrocyte sedimentation rate (ESR) or plasma viscosity;
- Labial gland biopsy;
- Other salivary studies (Table 5.2).

An oral rinse or swab should be taken to confirm the presence of candidiasis if there is soreness.

Management

Although it is desirable to control the underlying autoimmune disease, this is at present experimental only (e.g. cyclosporin). The patient should, however, be followed-up regularly, particularly because of the possible complication of lymphoma.

Table 5.2   Sjögren's syndrome: salivary studies

Investigation	Findings
Salivary flow rate (sialometry)	Reduced
Labial salivary gland biopsy	Focal lymphocytic infiltrate
	May help predict lymphomas
Scintiscanning (scintigraphy)	Reduced uptake of technetium
Sialography	Sialectasis

Other aspects of care include:

- Dry eyes: methylcellulose eye drops or rarely ligation or cautery of nasolacrimal duct. An ophthalmological opinion is indicated;
- Oral health care.

It is wise for the patient to avoid:

- Any drugs that may produce xerostomia (for example tricyclic antidepressants);
- Alcohol;
- Smoking;
- Dry foods such as biscuits.

Salivation may be stimulated by using:

- Chewing gums (containing sorbitol, not sucrose);
- Diabetic sweets;
- Cholinergic drugs that stimulate salivation (sialogogues), such as pilocarpine. These should be used by the specialist since they unfortunately may cause other cholinergic effects such as brady-cardia, sweating and the urge to urinate;
- Pyridostigmine is of greater benefit since it is longer-acting and associated with fewer adverse effects;
- Transglossal electrical stimulation;
- The lips should be protected with petroleum jelly;
- Salivary substitutes may help symptomatically (Table 10.10). Various are available including water, methylcellulose (Glandosane; Luborant; Saliveze; Salivace), a gel with lactoperoxidase, xylitol and glucose oxidase (Oralbelence), and mucin (Saliva Orthana). Olive oil may also help.

Dental caries

- Control of dietary sucrose intake;
- Daily use of fluorides (1% sodium fluoride gels or 0.4% stannous fluoride gels).

Candidiasis

- Dentures should be left out of the mouth at night and stored in sodium hypochlorite solution or chlorhexidine;
- An antifungal such as miconazole gel or amphotericin or nystatin ointment should be spread on the denture before re-insertion and a topical antifungal preparation, such as nystatin or amphotericin suspension, or lozenges used. Fluconazole is also effective.

Bacterial sialadenitis

Acute sialadenitis requires treatment with a penicillinase-resistant antibiotic such as flucloxacillin.

Xerostomia

See Chapter 1

Further reading

Chau MN, Radden BG. Intra-oral salivary gland neoplasms: a retrospective study of 98 cases. *J Oral Pathol* (1986) **15**: 339–42.

Di Alberti L, Piattelli A, Artese L et al. Human herpesvirus 8 variants in sarcoid tissues. *Lancet* (1997) **350**: 1655–61.

Epstein JB, Scully C. The role of saliva in oral health and the causes and effects of xerostomia. *J Can Dent Assoc* (1992) **58**: 217–21.

Epstein JB, Stevenson-Moore P, Scully C. Management of xerostomia. *J Can Dent Assoc* (1992) **58**: 140–3.

Eveson JW, Cawson RA. Salivary gland tumours. A review of 2410 cases with particular reference to histological types, site, age, and sex distribution. *J Pathol* (1985) **146**: 51–8.

Eveson JW, Scully C. *Colour Atlas of Oral Pathology.* (Mosby-Wolfe: London, 1995).

Jones JH, Mason DK. *Oral Manifestations of Systemic Disease*, 2nd edn. (Baillière: London, 1980).

Lamey PJ, Scully C. Diseases of the salivary glands. *Medicine International* (1990) **76**: 3167–9.

Main JH, Orr JA, McGurk FM et al. Salivary gland tumors: review of 643 cases. *J Oral Pathol* (1976) **5**: 88–102.

Mendelsohn SS, Field EA, Woolgar J. Sarcoidosis of the tongue. *Clin Exp Dermatol* (1992) **17**: 47–8.

Millard HD, Mason DK, eds. *Perspectives on 1993 World Workshop on Oral Medicine.* (University of Michigan: Ann Arbor, 1995).

Myer C, Cotton RT. Salivary gland disease in children: a review. *Clin Pediatr (Phila)* (1986) **25**: 314–22.

Porter SR, Scully C, eds. *Innovations and developments of non-surgical management of orofacial disease.* (Science Reviews: Northwood, 1996), pp. 1–229.

Scully C. Viruses and salivary gland disease. *Oral Surg Oral Med Oral Pathol* (1988) **66**: 179–83.

Scully C. Oral component of Sjogren's syndrome. In: Betail G, Sauvezie B, eds, *Le Syndrome de Gougerot Sjogren.* (Merck Sharp Dohme Chibret: Paris, 1991) 41–58.

Scully C. Non-neoplastic diseases of the major and minor salivary glands: a summary update. *Br J Oral Maxillofac Surg* (1992) **30**: 244–7.

Scully C, Cawson RA. *Medical Problems in Dentistry*, 4th edn. (Butterworth-Heinemann, Oxford, 1998).

Scully C, Porter SR. Oral Medicine: 3. Salivary disorders. *Postgrad Dent* (1993) **3**: 150–3.

Scully C, Welbury R. *Colour Atlas of Oral Disease in Children and Adolescents.* (Mosby-Wolfe: London, 1994).

Scully C, Flint S, Porter S. *Oral Diseases.* (Martin Dunitz: London, 1996).

Spiro RH. Salivary neoplasms: overview of a 35-year experience with 2807 patients. *Head Neck Surg* (1986) **8**: 177–84.

Van Maarsseveen ACMT, van der Waal I, Stam J et al. Oral involvement in sarcoidosis. *Int J Oral Surg* (1982) **11**: 21–9.

Vitali C, Bombardieri S, Moutsopoulos HM et al for the European Study Group on Diagnostic Criteria for Sjogren's Syndrome. Assessment of the European Classification criteria for Sjogren's syndrome in a series of clinically defined cases: results of a prospective multicentre study. *Ann Rheum Dis* (1996) **55**: 116–21.

6

Complaints particularly affecting gingivae

Bleeding

Most gingival bleeding is due to inflammatory gingival or periodontal disease (Figures 6.1, 6.6 and 6.15), sometimes exaggerated by hormonal changes such as pregnancy, but haemorrhagic disease (including leukaemia) (Figure 6.2) and drugs are occasionally responsible (Table 6.1).

Lumps and swellings

Discrete lumps (epulides) may be fibrous epulides, pyogenic granulomas, giant cell lesions or neoplasms. Generalized gingival swellings

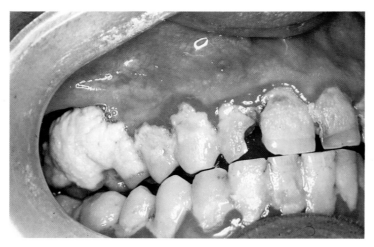

Figure 6.1
Gingival bleeding from marginal gingivitis and necrotizing gingivitis caused by appalling hygiene

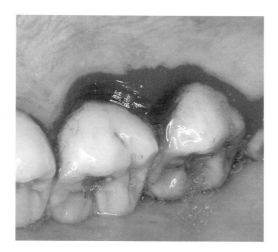

Figure 6.2
Gingival bleeding in leukaemia

Table 6.1   Causes of gingival bleeding

Local	Chronic gingivitis, chronic periodontitis, acute necrotizing gingivitis, telangiectasia, angioma
Systemic	Any thrombocytopathy, leukaemia, HIV infection, scurvy, clotting defects, drugs e.g. anticoagulants

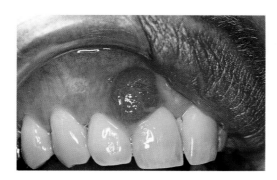

Figure 6.3
Pregnancy epulis (a pyogenic granuloma)

are sometimes congenital but most are due to hyperplasia with oedema related to plaque, occasionally exacerbated by hormonal changes (puberty, pregnancy) or drugs (Figures 6.3, 6.16 and 6.17).

Epulides

Epulides are localized gingival swellings.

Table 6.2   Main causes of gingival swelling

Multiple or generalized
  Local causes
    Chronic gingivitis, hyperplastic gingivitis due to mouth breathing
  Systemic causes
    Hereditary gingival fibromatosis and associated syndromes
    Drugs: phenytoin, cyclosporin, calcium channel blockers
    Granulomatous conditions: sarcoidosis, Crohn's disease, orofacial
    granulomatosis
    Leukaemia
    Scurvy
    Rare syndromes: Fabry's disease, Menke's disease, tuberose sclerosis,
    mucopolysaccharidoses, mucolipidosis, juvenile hyaline fibromatosis,
    lipoid proteinosis
    Plasma cell gingivostomatitis
    Infections: herpes simplex stomatis
    Neoplasms
    Wegener's granulomatosis
Localized
  Abscesses
  Cysts
  Warts
  Pyogenic granulomas including pregnancy epulis
  Neoplasms
  Wegener's granulomatosis

- Fibrous epulides: may result from local gingival irritation;
- Pyogenic granulomas: uncommon except as pregnancy epulides (lesions themselves not histologically distinguishable);
- Giant cell epulides: may result from proliferation of giant cells persisting after resorption of deciduous teeth;
- Rarely, epulides are carcinomas, Kaposi's sarcoma, lymphomas, metastases or other neoplasms.

Generalized gingival swelling (Table 6.2)

There are very few serious causes of generalized enlargements of gingivae appearing spontaneously or rapidly, but leukaemia is a prime suspect. Other gingival hyperplasias include Crohn's disease, sarcoidosis and orofacial granulomatosis. Infections that may cause gingival lesions include particularly herpetic stomatitis.

Red lesions

Most red lesions are inflammatory. Desquamative gingivitis, a common cause, is not a disease entity but a clinical term for persistently sore, glazed and red gingivae. It is fairly common, seen almost exclusively in middle-aged or elderly females and is usually a manifestation of atrophic lichen planus or mucous membrane pemphigoid (Figures 6.4 and 6.7). Other causes are shown in Table 6.3.

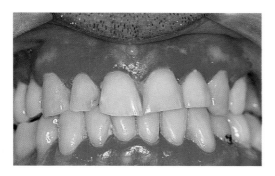

Figure 6.4
Desquamative gingivitis is usually caused by pemphigoid or lichen planus

Table 6.3   Causes of gingival redness

Gingivitis
   Inflammatory
   Desquamative
   Trauma
   Drugs
   Infections such as primary herpetic stomatitis
Granulomas
   Crohn's disease
   Orofacial granulomatosis
   Sarcoidosis
Erythroplasia
Plasma cell gingivostomatitis
Kaposi's sarcoma

Ulcers

Gingival ulcers are typical of necrotizing gingivitis and primary herpetic stomatitis but may be seen in other infections, especially in deep fungal infections, and may be caused by trauma, aphthae, malignant disease, skin diseases, haematological disorders, gastrointestinal disease and drugs.

Acute necrotizing ulcerative gingivitis (Vincent's disease)

Definition

Painful gingival papillary ulceration

Incidence

Uncommon

Age mainly affected

Young adults

Sex mainly affected

M>F

Aetiology

Acute ulcerative gingivitis (acute necrotizing ulcerative gingivitis, AUG, ANG, ANUG) is associated with proliferation of *Borrelia vincentii*, *Prevotella intermedia*, fusiform bacilli, selenomonas and other anaerobes. Predisposing factors include:

- Poor oral hygiene;
- Smoking;
- Malnutrition;
- Immune defects including HIV and other viral infections.

Clinical features

Features include the following:

- Painful ulceration of the interdental papillae which occasionally spreads to the gingival margins (see also cancrum oris) (Figure 6.5);
- A pronounced tendency to gingival bleeding;
- Halitosis;
- Sialorrhoea.

Diagnosis

Clinical features; smear

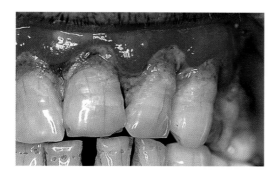

Figure 6.5
Acute necrotizing ulcerative gingivitis showing typical papillary ulceration

Management

- Oral debridement and hygiene instruction;
- Peroxide or perborate mouthwashes;
- Metronidazole (penicillin in pregnant females);
- Periodontal assessment.

Congenital epulis (granular cell myoblastoma)

Definition

Congenital epulis is a benign swelling on the alveolus in an infant.

Incidence

Rare

Age mainly affected

Infant

Sex mainly affected

F>M

Aetiology

Probably a reactive mesenchymal lesion arising from Schwann cells or pericytes, cells which stain for vimentin but not S100.

Clinical features

Congenital epulis is a benign tumour which usually presents:

- As a pedunculated firm pink swelling;
- <1 cm diameter;
- On the maxillary alveolus;
- In the canine region.

Diagnosis

Usually clinical but biopsy is confirmatory.

Management

It should be excised if there are feeding or breathing difficulties. The natural history may be of spontaneous regression.

Chronic hyperplastic gingivitis

Gingivitis may be hyperplastic, especially where there is mechanical irritation or mouth breathing, or sometimes it results from the use of some drugs (see page 283).

Chronic marginal gingivitis

Chronic marginal gingivitis is caused by the accumulation of dental plaque on the tooth close to the gingiva. Most of the adult population have a degree of gingivitis which commences in childhood. If plaque is not removed it calcifies to become calculus and this aggravates the condition by facilitating plaque accumulation. If left uncorrected, gingivitis may slowly and painlessly progress to periodontitis and ultimately to tooth loss.

Inflammation of the margins of the gingiva is painless and often the only features are:

- Gingival bleeding on brushing, or eating hard foods;
- Halitosis sometimes;
- Gingival erythema, swelling, and bleeding on examination (Figures 6.1, 6.6 and 6.15).

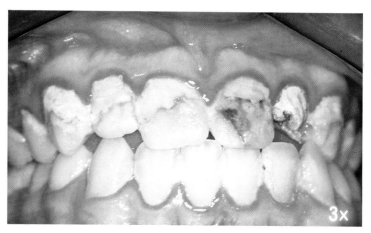

Figure 6.6
Chronic marginal gingivitis caused by poor oral hygiene

Desquamative gingivitis

Definition

Desquamative gingivitis is not a disease entity but a clinical term for persistently sore, glazed and red or ulcerated gingivae.

Incidence

Fairly common

Age mainly affected

Middle-aged or elderly

Sex mainly affected

F>M

Aetiology

Usually a manifestation of atrophic lichen planus (Figure 4.129) or mucous membrane pemphigoid (Figure 4.157), and occasionally seen in pemphigus or other dermatoses, desquamative gingivitis can also be due to chemicals or unknown causes.

Table 6.4   Main causes of desquamative gingivitis

Dermatoses	Pemphigoid, lichen planus, pemphigus, dermatitis herpetiformis, linear IgA disease
Chemicals	Sodium lauryl sulphate

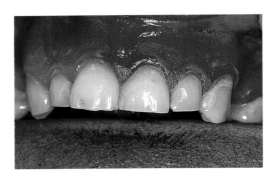

Figure 6.7
Desquamative gingivitis

Clinical features

The main features are:

- Persistent gingival soreness, worse on eating;
- Gingivae are red and glazed (patchily or uniformly) especially labially (Figures 6.4 and 6.7);
- Gingival erythema blurs the distinction between the normally coral pink attached gingivae and the more red vestibular mucosae;
- The erythema is exaggerated where oral hygiene is poor;
- Gingival margins and edentulous ridges tend to be spared;
- Other oral or cutaneous lesions of dermatoses may be associated.

Diagnosis

- The diagnosis is usually obvious from the history, with clinical findings, but other causes of red gingival lesions should be excluded (Table 6.3);
- Biopsy and immunostaining are often needed to establish the precise cause (Table 6.4).

Management

- Treatment should be of the underlying condition;
- Desquamative gingivitis can be improved if the oral hygiene is increased (Tables 10.1 and 10.2).

- Topical corticosteroids often help. Corticosteroid creams used overnight in a polythene splint are effective (Table 10.5);
- If there are extraoral lesions or severe oral ulceration in addition, systemic therapy, usually with corticosteroids may be required (Table 10.7);
- Other therapies available for recalcitrant desquamative gingivitis include cyclosporin, dapsone and tetracyclines.

Drug-induced gingival hyperplasia

Definition

Gingival swelling that occurs in response to the use of various drugs

Incidence

Common

Age mainly affected

Any

Sex mainly affected

M=F

Aetiology

The exact mechanism whereby the diverse drugs implicated act is unknown. All types of drug-induced gingival hyperplasia may also be associated with hirsutism. Drug-induced hyperplasia is usually worse where drug levels are high, and is aggravated by poor oral hygiene.

Clinical features

Phenytoin, a hydantoin anticonvulsant, is the drug that classically produces gingival hyperplasia, which appears interdentally 2–3 months after treatment is started. The gingival papillae enlarge to a variable extent, with relatively little tendency to bleed, and may even cover the tooth crowns (Figure 6.8). Hyperplasia peaks at around 1 year of drug use; it rarely affects edentulous areas. The hyperplasia is

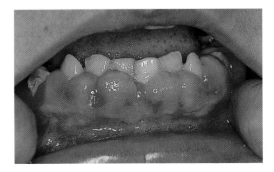

Figure 6.8
Phenytoin-induced gingival hyperplasia

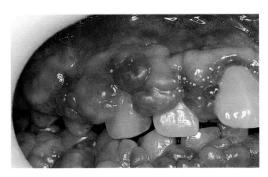

Figure 6.9
Cyclosporin-induced gingival hyperplasia

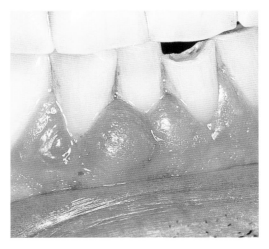

Figure 6.10
Nifedipine-induced gingival hyperplasia

proportional to the drug dose, though poor oral hygiene exacerbates the hyperplasia. Vigabatrin can produce a similar effect.

Cyclosporin, an immunosuppressive drug, can cause gingival hyperplasia closely resembling that induced by phenytoin (Figure 6.9). It is seen mainly anteriorly and labially and is exacerbated by poor oral hygiene and concurrent administration of nifedipine, but appears not to be proportional to the drug dose used.

Calcium channel blockers, dihydropyridines such as nifedipine, used as antihypertensives can produce gingival hyperplasia similar to that induced by phenytoin (Figure 6.10).

Diagnosis

Papillae are firm and pale, and enlarge to form false vertical clefts. Such changes often develop slowly, over weeks rather than days, and are usually painless.

Management

It may be possible to change or reduce the dose of the drug, in consultation with the physician. Otherwise, the oral hygiene should be improved and gingival surgery may be needed.

Fibrous epulis

Definition

The term epulis is applied to any lump arising from the gingiva. The fibrous epulis resembles a fibroepithelial polyp, but also usually has an inflammatory component.

Aetiology

Probably chronic irritation

Clinical features

The variable inflammatory changes account for the different clinical presentations from red, shiny and soft lumps to those that are pale, stippled and firm. Commonly they are round, painless, pedunculated swellings arising from the marginal or papillary gingiva, sometimes adjacent to sites of irritation (e.g. a carious cavity) (Figure 6.11); they rarely involve attached gingiva, and rarely exceed 2 cm in diameter.

Diagnosis and management

The diagnosis is clinical, confirmed by excision biopsy.

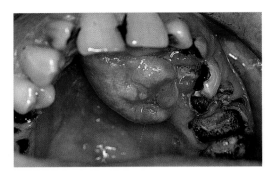

Figure 6.11
Fibrous epulis

Giant cell granuloma (giant cell epulis; peripheral giant cell granuloma)

Definition

This is a non-neoplastic swelling of proliferating fibroblasts in a highly vascular stroma containing many multinucleate giant cells.

Incidence

Uncommon

Age mainly affected

Children

Sex mainly affected

F>M

Aetiology

The resorption of deciduous teeth and remodelling of the alveolus at the mixed dentition stage indicate the osteoclastic potential of the area from which giant cell epulides arise. The lesion probably arises because chronic irritation triggers a reactionary hyperplasia of mucoperiosteum and excessive production of granulation tissue. Giant cell granulomas, unless they are extraosseous, may also be a feature of hyperparathyroidism.

Clinical features

The giant cell epulis characteristically (Figure 6.12):

- Is notable for the deep-red or purple colour, although older lesions tend to be paler;
- Arises interdentally;
- Is seen adjacent to permanent teeth which have had predecessors, so is seen anterior to the permanent molars;
- Is a benign lesion.

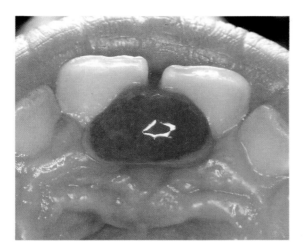

Figure 6.12
Giant cell epulis

Diagnosis

- Biopsy is usually required;
- The area should be examined radiographically;
- To exclude hyperparathyroidism, levels of plasma calcium, phosphate and alkaline phosphatase should be assayed.

Management

Treatment depends on the cause. If hyperparathyroidism is present, this must be treated. Treatment otherwise is surgical. The lesion may recur.

Gingival cysts in neonates

Small white nodules sometimes termed Epstein's pearls or Bohn's nodules, are extremely common on the alveolar ridge and midline palate of the newborn. They usually disappear spontaneously by rupturing or involution within a month or so. There may be an association with milia (superficial epidermal inclusion cysts).

Hereditary gingival fibromatosis

Definition

Hereditary gingival fibromatosis is a familial condition, in which there is generalized gingival fibromatosis.

Incidence

Uncommon

Age mainly affected

From childhood

Sex mainly affected

M=F

Aetiology

Autosomal dominant condition

Clinical features

- The family history is typically positive;
- The condition presents as generalized gingival enlargement, especially obvious during the transition from deciduous to permanent dentition;
- The changes involve the papillae and later the attached gingiva, and, if the enlargement is gross, it may move or cover the teeth and bulge out of the mouth;
- The affected gingiva is usually of normal colour but firm in consistency, and the surface, although initially smooth, becomes coarsely stippled (Figure 6.13);
- Gingival hyperplasia is often associated with hirsutism;

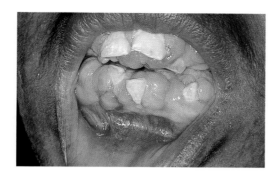

Figure 6.13
Hereditary gingival fibromatosis

- There are occasional associations with epilepsy, sensorineural deafness and some rare syndromes such as Laband syndrome (in which there are skeletal anomalies).

Diagnosis

Diagnosis is clinical.

Management

Surgery is often indicated.

Lateral periodontal abscess (parodontal abscess)

Definition

An abscess arising in a periodontal pocket

Incidence

Uncommon

Age mainly affected

Adults

Sex mainly affected

M=F

Aetiology

Lateral periodontal abscesses:

- Are seen almost exclusively in patients with chronic periodontitis;
- May follow impaction of a foreign body;
- Are rarely related to a lateral root canal on a nonvital tooth.

Debris and pus cannot escape easily from the pocket and therefore an abscess results.

Clinical features

Lateral periodontal abscesses usually present with:

- Pain;
- Swelling.

They discharge either through the pocket or buccally, but more coronally than a periapical abscess.

Diagnosis

Clinical

Management

Establish drainage, usually by curettage.

Papillon–Lefevre syndrome

Definition

Papillon–Lefevre syndrome is a genetically linked disorder manifesting with prepubertal periodontitis in association with palmar–plantar hyperkeratosis and sometimes an immune defect.

Incidence

Rare

Age mainly affected

Childhood

Sex mainly affected

M=F

Aetiology

Genetic defect in cathepsin

Clinical features

- Tooth loss: virtually all primary teeth are involved and most are lost by the age of 4 years. The permanent teeth are often lost by the age of 16 years;
- Hyperkeratosis usually affects the soles more severely than the palms;
- The dura mater may be calcified, particularly the tentorium. The choroid can also be calcified.

A rare variant of the Papillon–Lefevre syndrome includes arachno-dactyly and tapered phalanges as well as the above features.

Diagnosis

Clinical features

Management

Retinoids may help.

Pericoronitis

Definition

Inflammation of the operculum over an erupting or impacted tooth

Incidence

Common

Age mainly affected

Adolescents and teenagers

Sex mainly affected

M=F

Aetiology

Accumulation of plaque/debris beneath an operculum, and irritation by an occluding tooth

Clinical features

The lower third molar is the site most commonly affected (Figure 6.14) but it is occasionally seen in relation to second molars. Patients complain of:

- Pain;
- Trismus;
- Swelling of the operculum;
- Halitosis.

In **acute** pericoronitis, there may also be:

- Swollen, red and often ulcerated operculum;
- Pus from beneath operculum;
- Some facial swelling;
- Fever;
- Regional lymphadenitis;
- Malaise.

Diagnosis

Clinical features

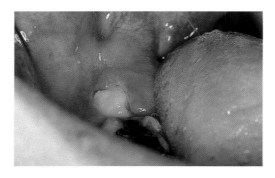

Figure 6.14
Pericoronitis

Management

- Remove any irritation by an occluding tooth cusp;
- Irrigate the opercular region with saline;
- Possibly apply astringent such as trichloracetic acid to the under-surface of the operculum;
- Give antimicrobials such as metronidazole or penicillin if there are systemic symptoms/signs;
- Consider removal of the offending tooth after acute features have subsided.

Periodontitis

Definition

Inflammatory-mediated destruction of alveolar bone support, with deep pocket formation and associated tooth mobility and migration

Incidence

Common

Age mainly affected

Adults

Sex mainly affected

M=F

Aetiology

- Typically related to plaque accumulation;
- Periodontitis may rarely develop where there is good control of plaque and is then typically related to an immune defect which may be acquired or inherited:
  - Accelerated (prepubertal) periodontitis is a rare condition seen in children;
  - Localized juvenile periodontitis is characterized by localized periodontal destruction, classically in the permanent incisor

and first molar regions in adolescent or young adults in the absence of poor oral hygiene or gross systemic disease;

- Juvenile periodontitis (periodontosis) is seen especially in females, and may be associated with minor defects of neutrophil function and with microorganisms such as *Actinobacillus actinomycetemcomitans* and *capnocytophaga*;
- Papillon–Lefevre syndrome, Down's syndrome, type VIII Ehlers–Danlos syndrome and hypophosphatasia;
- Poorly controlled diabetes mellitus, white cell dyscrasias including neutrophil defects and neutropenias, and other immune defects including HIV/AIDS.

Clinical features

The features are those of marginal gingivitis but, with destruction of alveolar bone support (Figures 6.1 and 6.15), there is:

- Deep pocket formation;
- Tooth mobility and migration;
- Halitosis.

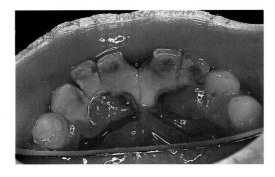

Figure 6.15
Chronic periodontitis

Diagnosis

Clinical and radiographical

Management

- Oral hygiene;
- Scaling and root planing;
- Periodontal surgery.

Peripheral odontogenic fibroma

This is a rare benign reactive condition seen mainly in Blacks and on the gingiva. It consists of mineralized tissue that resembles dentine, cementum or osteoid, may erode bone or displace teeth and should be excised.

Plasma cell gingivitis (idiopathic circumorificial plasmacytosis)

This is an uncommon erythematous and oedematous reaction to substances such as:

- Chewing gum;
- Cinnamonaldehyde;
- Cinnamon oil;
- Dichlorophene;
- Foods;
- Hexylresorcinol;
- Mint.

A careful history is required, concentrating on exposure to chewing gum or oral medications. Patch tests on the skin are usually negative. The offending substance should be withdrawn.

Pregnancy gingivitis and pregnancy epulis

Definition

Gingivitis or epulis in pregnancy

Incidence

Common mainly after 2nd month of pregnancy

Age mainly affected

Adult

Sex affected

F

Aetiology

Poor oral hygiene predisposes to exacerbation of chronic gingivitis as a result of increased progestogen levels. Changes appear first around the second month of pregnancy, reach a peak at the eighth month and may revert to the previous level of gingival health soon after parturition.

Clinical features

Pregnancy gingivitis (Figure 6.16) is characterized by:

- Soft, reddish enlargements;
- Usually of the gingival papillae;
- Mainly labial location of swelling;
- Gingival bleeding, particularly on eating or toothbrushing.

Pregnancy epulis (epulis gravidarum; Figures 6.3 and 6.17) is:

- A localized gingival lump;
- Typically located on a labial interdental papilla.

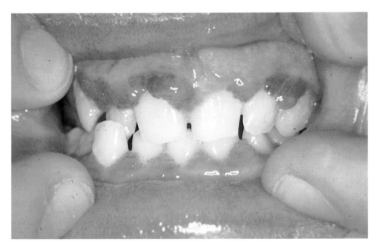

Figure 6.16
Pregnancy gingivitis (the fingers are the patient's)

Diagnosis

- Clinical features and history;
- Pregnancy test occasionally;
- Biopsy rarely.

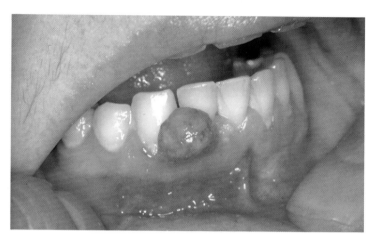

Figure 6.17
Pregnancy epulis

Management

Pregnancy gingivitis: Oral hygiene.
Pregnancy epulis: Conservative treatment is indicated unless an epulis interferes with occlusion or is extremely unsightly when it can be excised. In any event, oral hygiene should be meticulous.

Retrocuspid papilla

An anatomical variant found on the lingual gingiva in the mandibular canine region. It resembles the incisive papilla.

Scurvy

Definition

Swollen gingivae and petechiae from vitamin C deficiency

Incidence

Rare

Age mainly affected

Adults

Sex mainly affected

M=F

Aetiology

Vitamin C (ascorbic acid) deficiency. The condition results when no fresh fruit or vegetables are eaten for a long period.

Clinical features

Lesions include:

- **Gingivae**: diffusely swollen, boggy, and purplish with purpura and haemorrhage;
- **Skin**: perifollicular haemorrhages.

Diagnosis

- The diagnosis is clear from the dietary history and clinical features;
- The classic investigation is assay of white cell ascorbic acid.

Management

- Give vitamin C (ascorbic acid) supplements;
- Reform the diet.

Tuberose sclerosis (epiloia or Bourneville disease)

This is a rare autosomal dominant condition in which there may be:

- Enamel pitting hypoplasia;
- Gingival swellings;
- Cortical hyperostosis and sometimes pseudocystic radiolucencies in the mandible;
- Skin lesions of various types, especially angiofibromas;
- Fibromas at the nail bed (subungual fibromas or Koenen's tumours);
- Epilepsy;
- Sometimes learning disability.

Further reading

Bakaeen G, Scully C. Hereditary gingival fibromatosis in a family with the Zimmermann–Laband syndrome. *J Oral Pathol Med* (1991) **20**: 457–9.

Cianco S, Rees T, Meiders M et al. Consensus report. Periodontal implications: mucocutaneous disorders. *Ann Periodontol* (1996) **1**: 439–42.

Clark D. Gingival fibromatosis and related syndromes. *J Can Dent Assoc* (1987) **6**: 137–40.

Porter SR, Scully C. Periodontal aspects of systemic disease. A system of classification. In: Lang N, ed., *European Workshop of Periodontology.* (Quintessence: Berlin, 1994), 374–419.

Porter SR, Scully C. Periodontal aspects of systemic disease. Some therapeutic concepts. In: Lang N, ed., *European Workshop of Periodontology.* (Quintessence: Berlin, 1994) 415–38.

Porter SR, Scully C, Mutlu S. Viral infections affecting periodontal health. *Periodont Clin Invest* (1995) **15**: 17–24.

Scully C. Diagnosis and diagnostic procedures: general and soft tissue diagnosis. In: *Pathways in Practice* (Faculty of General Dental Practice, Royal College of Surgeons of England: City, 1993) 25–33.

Scully C. The pathology of orofacial disease. In: Barnes IE, Walls AWG, eds, *Gerodontology* (Wright-Butterworths: Oxford, 1994) 29–41.

Scully C. Prevention of oral mucosal disease. In: Murray JJ, ed., *Prevention of Oral and Dental Disease*, 3rd edn. (Oxford University Press: Oxford, 1995) 160–72.

Scully C. The oral cavity. In: Champion RH, Burton J, Burns DA, Breathnach SM, eds, *Textbook of Dermatology*, 5th edn (Blackwells: Oxford, 1998) 3047–123.

Scully C, Cawson RA. *Medical Problems in Dentistry*, 4th edn. (Butterworth-Heinemann: Oxford, 1998).

Scully C, Porter SR. Disorders of the gums and periodontium. *Med Int* (1990) **76**: 3150–3.

Scully C, Porter SR. Oral medicine: 1. Teeth and periodontium. *Postgrad. Dent* (1992) **2**: 93–100.

Scully C, Porter SR. Oral mucosal disease: a decade of new entities, aetiologies and associations. *Int Dent J* (1994) **44**: 33–43.

Scully C, Welbury R. *Colour Atlas of Oral Disease in Children and Adolescents.* (Mosby-Wolfe: London, 1994).

Scully C, Porter SR, Mutlu S. Markers of disease susceptibility and activity for periodontal diseases: changing subject-based risk factors. In: Johnson NW, ed., *Risk Markers for Oral Disease: 3. Periodontal Diseases.* (Cambridge University Press: Cambridge, 1991) 139–78.

Scully C, Flint S, Porter S. *Oral Diseases* (Martin Dunitz: London, 1996).

Seymour RA, Jacobs DJ. Cyclosporin and the gingival tissues. *J Clin Periodontol* (1992) **19**: 1–11.

7

Lip complaints

The lips mainly consist of bundles of striated muscle, particularly the orbicularis oris muscle, with skin on the external surface and mucous membrane on the inner surface, which has a profusion of minor salivary glands.

The lips extend from the lower end of the nose to the upper chin. The upper lip includes the philtrum, a midline depression, extending from the columella of the nose to the superior edge of the vermilion zone. The oral commissures are the angles where the upper and lower lip meet.

The vermilion zone, the transitional zone between the glabrous skin and the mucous membrane, is found only in humans. The vermilion zone contains no hair or sweat glands but frequently contains sebaceous glands (Fordyce spots: Chapter 4). The epithelium of the vermilion is distinctive, with a prominent stratum lucidum and a very thin stratum corneum. The dermal papillae there are numerous, with a rich capillary supply, which produces the reddish-pink colour of the lips in Caucasians. Melanocytes are abundant in the basal layer of the vermilion of pigmented skin, but are infrequent in Caucasian skin.

Bleeding

Lips may bleed because of:

- Trauma;
- Fissures;
- Erythema multiforme;
- Angiomas;
- Telangiectases;
- Haemorrhagic disease (Figure 7.1).

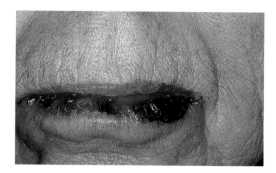

Figure 7.1
Bleeding into herpetic lesions in a leukaemic with thrombocytopenia

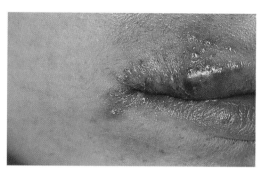

Figure 7.2
Recurrent herpes labialis

Blisters

Blisters on the lips may be caused by:

- Herpes labialis (Figures 7.2, 7.24, 7.25 and 4.90–4.92) but other less common causes include:
- Burns;
- Mucoceles;
- Impetigo;
- Allergic cheilitis;
- Herpes zoster;
- Erythema multiforme;
- Pemphigus;
- Drugs, especially fixed drug eruption;
- Epidermolysis bullosa.

Chapping

Chapping is usually a reaction to adverse environmental conditions:

- Exposure to cold or hot dry winds;

- Fever;
- Dehydration;
- Cheilitis;
- Erythema multiforme;
- Psychogenic causes;
- Drugs.

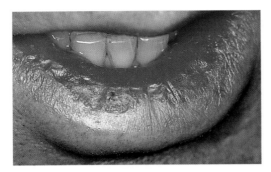

Figure 7.3
Chapped lips

The lips, especially the lower, become sore, cracked and scaly (Figure 7.3). The affected subject tends to lick the lips, or to pick at the scales, which may make the condition worse. Petroleum jelly applications help, as does avoidance of the causative conditions.

Cheilitis (inflammation of the lips)

Cheilitis may be caused by various factors (Table 7.1) including:

- Lip-licking habits (tic de levres); may lead to cheilitis and erythematous circumoral lesions;

Table 7.1   Causes of cheilitis

Allergies (e.g. to lipstick)	Glandular cheilitis
Chapping due to cold and wind	Granulomatous cheilitis
Eczematous cheilitis	Exfoliative (factitious) cheilitis
Chemical or other burns	Plasma cell cheilitis
Contact cheilitis	Nutritional cheilitis
Drug-induced cheilitis (e.g. etretinate)	Dermatoses
Infective cheilitis	Trauma
Angular cheilitis	Kawasaki disease
Ultraviolet irradiation:	
Actinic cheilitis	
Actinic prurigo of the lip	

- Exfoliative cheilitis; this is persistent scaling of the vermilion of the lips, seen mainly in adolescent or young adult females, often in a somewhat cyclical nature. It is of unknown, possibly factitious, aetiology. The lips scale and peel and can be covered with a shaggy yellowish coating.

Candidiasis may infect these lesions.

Coloured lesions

Coloured lesions are usually innocuous conditions such as Fordyce spots or melanotic macules but they may also signify more serious disease such as Kaposi's sarcoma (Table 7.2).

- In some people sebaceous glands (Fordyce spots) may be seen as creamy-yellow dots along the border between the vermilion and the oral mucosa;
- Red or purple lesions may be telangiectases, angiomas, Kaposi's sarcoma or epithelioid angiomatosis;
- Brown lesions are usually melanotic. The labial melanotic macule is an acquired small, flat, brown to brown-black asymptomatic benign lesion. Peutz–Jegher's syndrome may present with multiple melanotic macules. Some other syndromes and drugs cause hyper-pigmentation (Table 7.2).

Table 7.2   Pigmented lesions of the lips

Melasma
Melanotic macule
Smoker's melanosis
Naevi
Pigmented neuroectodermal tumour
Mucocutaneous pigmented spots and oral myxomas
Peutz–Jegher syndrome
Laugier–Hunziker–Baran syndrome
Lupus pernio
Ephelis
Lentigo simplex
Solar lentigo
Carney syndrome
Tattoos
Addison's disease
Albright's syndrome
Drugs (e.g. zidovudine, contraceptive pill)
Heavy metal poisoning

Desquamation and crusting

See Cheilitis

Macrostomia

Macrostomia is uncommon but may be seen in:
- Facioauriculovertebral syndrome;
- Mucopolysaccharidoses;
- Beckwith–Wiedemann syndrome.

Generalized swelling of the lips may be seen in
- Trauma;
- Infection;
- Erythema multiforme;
- Angioedema;
- Orofacial granulomatosis;
- Crohn's disease;
- Sarcoidosis;
- Melkersson–Rosenthal syndrome;
- Cheilitis glandularis;
- Lymphangioma;
- Haemangioma;
- Plasma cell orificial mucositis;
- Extramedullary plasmacytoma;
- Ascher's syndrome;
- Mucopolysaccharidoses;
- Fucosidosis;
- Coffin–Siris syndrome;
- Liptip syndrome.

Table 7.3   Causes of swelling of the lip

Inflammatory	Infections, bites, Crohn's disease, orofacial granulomatosis, sarcoidosis
Traumatic	Traumatic or postoperative surgical emphysema
Immunologically mediated	Angioedema
Endocrine and metabolic	Obesity, systemic corticosteroid therapy, Cushing's syndrome, myxoedema, acromegaly, nephrotic syndrome, cysts, hamartomas, neoplasms.

Localized swellings may be due to:
- Trauma;
- Orofacial granulomatosis;
- Crohn's disease;
- Sarcoidosis;
- Melkersson–Rosenthal syndrome;
- Mucoceles;
- Pyogenic granuloma;
- Cysts;
- Abscesses;
- Insect bites;
- Haematomas;
- Sucking pads (calluses);
- Chancre;
- Salivary adenoma;
- Squamous cell carcinoma;
- Basal cell carcinoma;
- Keratoacanthoma;
- Other tumours;
- Cowden's syndrome.

Microstomia

The size of the oral opening has wide individual variability. Diminution of the oral opening (microstomia) can result from:
- Scarring, for example from burns;
- Systemic sclerosis;
- Oral submucous fibrosis;
- Congenital conditions including: cranio-carpotarsal syndrome, otopalatal digital syndrome, Hallerman–Streiff syndrome, Robinous syndrome.

White lesions

White lesions of the lips are usually keratoses from smoking or sun-exposure, or lichen planus. Causes include:
- Keratoses;
- Actinic keratosis;
- Carcinoma;
- Lichen planus;
- Lupus erythematosus;
- Candidiasis;
- Scars;

- Fordyce spots;
- Various congenital conditions.

Abnormal labial fraenum

A labial maxillary fraenum may occasionally be associated with a maxillary median diastema-spacing between the central incisors. The fraenum may need to be removed before the diastema can be closed by orthodontic means.

Actinic cheilitis (actinic keratosis of lip; solar cheilosis)

Definition

A premalignant keratosis of the lip caused by exposure to solar irradiation

Incidence

Common in sunny climes, especially in caucasians

Age mainly affected

Middle-aged and elderly

Sex mainly affected

M>F

Aetiology

Cheilitis due to acute sunburn is common, and clinically resembles 'chapping'. Actinic cheilitis is most common in hot, dry regions, in outdoor workers and in fair-skinned people. Other forms of radiation including arc-welding can cause similar changes.

Clinical features

Acute cheilitis is characterized by erythema, oedema and soreness followed by scaling (Figures 4.36 and 7.4).

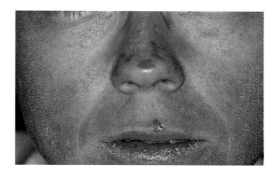

Figure 7.4
Actinic burns on the nose and lip and cheilitis

Chronic actinic cheilitis is characterized by atrophy and eventually keratosis, mainly over the entire lower lip. Erosions or induration may herald carcinomatous change which affects up to 10%.

Diagnosis

* The diagnosis is clinical and the history is usually helpful;
* Biopsy may be warranted in chronic cheilitis or where there are erosions or induration.

The possibility of malignant change must always be considered when there are suspect features such as:

* Ulceration or erosions;
* Red and white blotchy appearance with an indistinct vermilion border;
* Generalized atrophy with focal areas of whitish thickening;
* Persistent flaking and crusting.

The histology shows a flattened or atrophic epithelium, beneath which is a band of inflammatory infiltrate in which plasma cells may predominate. Nuclear atypia and abnormal mitoses may be seen in the more severe cases, and some develop into invasive squamous carcinoma. The collagen generally shows basophilic (elastotic) degeneration.

Management

* Adequate sunscreens (liquid or gel waterproof preparations) are needed in those with high exposure to UVB, such as mountaineers, sailors and skiers, and in patients with rare photosensitivity disorders such as xeroderma pigmentosum;
* Treatment to relieve symptoms and to prevent development of squamous carcinoma includes applications two to three times

daily for 10–14 days of 5-fluorouracil, or tretinoin or trichloracetic acid;
- Vermilionectomy (lip shave) or carbon dioxide laser ablation for premalignant or malignant lesions.

Angioedema

Definition

Acute diffuse swelling of the lips and/or face

Incidence

Rare

Age mainly affected

Any

Sex mainly affected

M=F

Aetiology

There are two main types.

Allergic angioedema

Allergic angioedema (a type 1 hypersensitivity response) is the most common form of angioedema and is idiopathic in 90% of cases, but also occurs in relation to contact with an antigen such as a food or drug.

- **Foods**: eggs, nuts, chocolate, fish, strawberries, milk, peaches, spices, pork, yeast;
- **Bites/stings**;
- **Drugs**: angiotensin converting enzyme inhibitors, captopril, antihypertensives, antibiotics, NSAIDs, doxorubicin, opiates, sedatives, vaccines, aspirin, carbamazepine, barbiturates, chlorpromazine, dextran.

Urticaria may be associated with angioedema. Oedema may involve the lips, buccal mucosa, tongue and uvula.

Hereditary angioneurotic oedema

HANE: caused by a deficiency of the inhibitor of C1 esterase, when the swelling occurs in response to trauma or stress. Oedema may involve the lips, buccal mucosa, tongue and uvula. Attacks are painless but the oedema may threaten the airway and the mortality rate is high in some families. There is no urticaria. Attacks generally subside within 24 hours. There may be associated abdominal pain.

This is usually an autosomal dominant condition appearing in childhood and worsening in adolescence. It may also occasionally arise in B cell lymphoproliferative diseases (chronic lymphocytic leukaemia, plasmacytoma, lymphoma) as an autoimmune disorder.

Clinical features

Swelling of the lips in angioedema is characterized by:

* Acute onset;
* Relatively transient nature of the swelling (<72 hours);
* Nonpitting oedema;
* Painless usually;
* A lack of scaling (Figure 7.5);
* Usually affecting the whole lip(s), sometimes the face, neck and elsewhere.

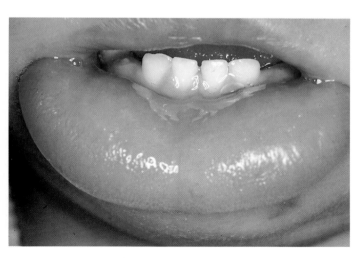

Figure 7.5
Angioedema: diffuse swelling of lip

The angioedema is often mild but there is always the potential for obstruction of the airway.

Diagnosis

- The diagnosis is usually clinical with acute swelling typically related to administration of a drug, or in the case of HANE, related to trauma or stress;
- There may be a family history of HANE;
- Serum levels of C2, C4 and C1 esterase inhibitor should be assessed in order to exclude HANE. All are reduced in HANE.

Management

- The airway must be maintained;
- It may be necessary to give oxygen;
- **Allergic angioedema** is treated with intramuscular adrenaline, and with corticosteroids and antihistamines;
- **Hereditary angioedema** is treated with C1 esterase inhibitor concentrate, stanazolol, or fresh frozen plasma.

Angular cheilitis (angular stomatitis)

Definition

Angular stomatitis is an acute or chronic inflammation of the skin and contiguous labial mucous membrane at the angles of the mouth.

Incidence

Common

Age mainly affected

Elderly

Sex mainly affected

M=F

Aetiology

Angular stomatitis is a common clinical syndrome, in which may be implicated:

- infective agents;
- mechanical factors;
- immune deficiency; or
- nutritional deficiencies.

Most cases in adults are due to mechanical and/or infective causes but nutritional or immune defects are more prominent causes in children.

Mechanical factors

In the edentulous patient who does not wear a denture or who has inadequate dentures, the upper lip overhangs the lower at the angles of the mouth, producing an oblique curved fold and keeping a small area of skin constantly macerated.

Infective agents

Oral candidiasis causing stomatitis is particularly common in those wearing dentures. Staphylococci appear to infect from the anterior nares.

Immune deficiency

Angular stomatis associated with candidiasis resistant to therapy may be an early manifestation of an underlying immune deficiency such as diabetes and HIV disease.

Nutritional deficiencies

Deficiencies of riboflavin, folate, iron and general protein malnutrition have often been incriminated.

Salivary factors

Hypersalivation from any cause may ensure the continued maceration of the angles of the mouth, but xerostomia is a more common cause since it predisposes to candidiasis.

Clinical features

Angular cheilitis presents:

- As a roughly triangular area of erythema and oedema at the commissures (Figures 7.6 and 7.7);
- Commonly at both angles of the mouth (Figures 7.8 and 7.9);
- Linear furrows or fissures radiating from the angle of the mouth (rhagades) are seen in the more severe forms, especially in denture wearers;
- Recurrent exudation and crusting are frequent.

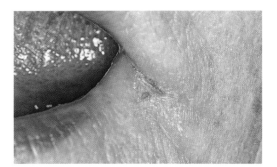

Figure 7.6
Angular stomatitis:
typical appearance

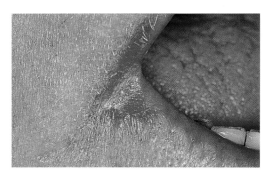

Figure 7.7
Angular stomatitis:
fissuring and soreness

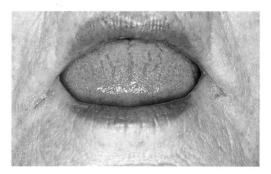

Figure 7.8
Angular stomatitis:
typically a bilateral
condition

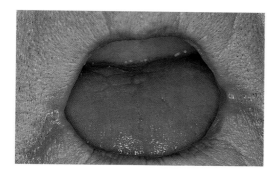

Figure 7.9
*Angular stomatitis:
typically seen with
chronic atrophic
candidiasis (denture-
induced stomatis)*

Diagnosis

- This is usually clinically obvious;
- Diabetes and anaemia should be excluded. May need blood picture, blood glucose, smears for fungal hyphae, microbiological culture;
- Candida should be sought in denture wearers, not only in the lesions but also beneath the denture, by swabbing palate and denture, and taking an oral rinse;
- Rare mimics include acanthosis nigricans, acrodermatitis enteropathica, glucagonoma and pemphigus vegetans.

Management

- Underlying systemic disease must be sought and treated especially in the young, dentate or where there is unilateral stomatitis;
- Reducing the sugar content of the diet may help reduce candida counts;
- Acrylic dentures should be kept out of the mouth as much as possible and stored at night for at least 2 weeks in a candidacidal solution such as hypochlorite. Metal dentures may discolour in hypochlorite, and thus chlorhexidine should be used;
- Antifungal cream (usually miconazole) should be applied to the lesions of angular stomatitis, several times daily. This is the preferable treatment (cream applied locally, together with oral gel to treat denture-induced stomatitis) as it has some Gram-positive bacteriostatic action. However, there is a high relapse rate unless treatment is prolonged. Miconazole is absorbed and may potentiate the action of warfarin, phenytoin and the sulphonylurea. Nystatin or amphotericin (as cream of ointment) should therefore be tried first in patients taking these drugs. Fluconazole is also effective;

- Denture-induced stomatitis should be treated with an antifungal;
- The nares and skin lesions should be swabbed and staphylococcal infection treated with fusidic acid ointment or cream at least four times daily;
- New dentures which restore facial contour may help;
- In rare intractable cases, a course of oral iron and vitamin B supplements may be helpful, but surgery or occasionally collagen injections may be needed to try to restore normal commissural anatomy.

Carcinoma of the lip

Definition

Squamous carcinoma

Incidence

Uncommon

Age mainly affected

Middle aged and elderly

Sex mainly affected

M>F

Aetiology

Risk factors may include:
- Actinic damage. Like actinic cheilitis it is most common on the lower lip of fair-skinned outdoor workers in sunny climates, and it is relatively rare in pigmented skin. Lip cancer generally occurs in men who are employed in outdoor activities such as farming and fishing;
- Low social class;
- Tobacco smoking;
- Infection with herpes simplex virus;
- Immune suppression.

Clinical features

The initial features are swelling of the lip with induration (Figure 7.10), soreness and ulceration. Squamous cancers of the lip occur on the lower lip in 89% with 3% on the upper lip and 8% at the commissures. Most occur on the mucocutaneous junction. Cervical lymph node enlargement should be excluded as this may represent metastases.

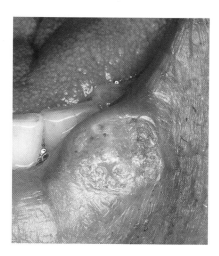

Figure 7.10
Carcinoma of the lip: an indurated swelling at the typical site

Diagnosis

Biopsy is required to confirm the diagnosis.

Management

Most lesions are amenable to surgical excision, with more than 70% surviving for 5 years.

Cheilitis glandularis

Definition

Cheilitis glandularis is a chronic inflammatory disorder of minor salivary glands in which there is hypersecretion and ductal ectasia.

Incidence

Rare

Age mainly affected

Adults

Sex mainly affected

M>F

Aetiology

Idiopathic but risk factors may include actinic damage. Like actinic cheilitis it is most common on the lower lip and it is possible that the everted mucosa develops a compensatory hyperplasia to protect itself, resulting in ductal ectasia and metaplasia.

Clinical features

The lower lip is usually affected and appears:
- Swollen;
- Everted;
- To show superficial puncta of the salivary ducts as red, white or black dots;
- To exude a thick sticky substance that may form a crust on the lip.

Cheilitis glandularis has been associated with squamous cell carcinoma.

Diagnosis

- Clinical;
- Biopsy.

Management

- There is no specific treatment;
- Symptomatic relief may be obtained from lip balms, sunscreens, antihistamines, corticosteroids or antibiotics;
- If the above fail, cryosurgery or vermilionectomy may be effective;

- Because of the risk of carcinoma, surgery is needed in advanced disease.

Cleft lip and palate

Definition

Incomplete fusion of facial growth processes

Incidence

Cleft lip and/or palate are the most common congenital craniofacial abnormalities and affect about 1 per 1000 births.

Age mainly affected

From birth

Sex mainly affected

M=F

Aetiology

- There is familial tendency when one parent is affected, and the risk to a child is about 10%;
- Cleft lip appears reduced if women take multivitamins containing folic acid early in pregnancy;
- Many cases are associated with various syndromes.

Clinical features

Cleft lip is not always complete (i.e. extending into the nostril). A cleft may involve only the upper lip or may extend to involve the nostril and the hard and soft palates. Isolated cleft lip may be unilateral or bilateral (approximately 20%). Lips are more frequently cleft bilaterally (approximately 25%) when combined with cleft palate. Clefts in the middle of the upper lip may be true or false. True median clefts have been described in association with bifid nose and ocular hypertelorism. Other cases of true median labial cleft are associated with polydactyly or other digital anomalies, constituting an autosomal recessive trait called the orofaciodigital syndrome. Pseudocleft of the middle of the upper lip may occur in orofaciodigital syndrome I. Clefts in the lower lip are rare and usually median but may involve the mandible and sometimes the tongue.

Bifid or cleft uvula is a fairly common minor manifestation of cleft palate but of little consequence, though an associated submucous cleft may cause speech impairment. Cleft lip and palate are more common together than is cleft lip alone. The cleft is on the left in over 60% of patients.

Cleft lip and palate are, in about 20% of cases, associated with anomalies of head and neck, extremities, genitalia or heart. Clefts are often accompanied by impaired facial growth, dental anomalies, speech disorders, poor hearing and psychosocial problems.

The **Robin syndrome** (or sequence, Pierre–Robin syndrome) is:

- Severe congenital micrognathia with cleft palate:
- There may be glossoptosis and respiratory embarrassment;
- Episodic dyspnoea is often evident from birth;
- There may also be congenital cardiac anomalies and, rarely, learning disability.

The Robin sequence may be seen in:

- Stickler syndrome (a disorder of type II collagen);
- fetal alcohol syndrome;
- fetal methodone syndrome;
- fetal epanutin syndrome.

Contact cheilitis

Definition

Contact cheilitis is an inflammatory reaction of the lips, provoked by the irritant or sensitizing action of chemical agents.

Incidence

Uncommon

Age mainly affected

Any age but predominantly adults

Sex mainly affected

F>M

Table 7.4   Items sometimes causing contact cheilitis

Dentifrices/mouthwashes	Aniseed oil, clove oil, ethylene diamine, menthol, parabens, pimento oil, pyrophosphate, tromantadine
Foods	Apples, artichokes, lemons, mangoes, oranges
Lip balm allergens	Antibiotics, phenyl salicylate
Lipstick allergens	Antioxidants, azo dyes, azulene, carmine, cinnamon, colophony, eosin, fluorescein, lanolin, peppermint, perfumes, preservatives, propyl gallate, sesame oil, shellac, spearmint
Nail polish	Formaldehyde
Others	Pens, pencils, pins

Aetiology

Many substances have been incriminated (Table 7.4), but most cases are caused by cosmetics or foods. Causes include:

- Tartar control dentifrices;
- Dental materials;
- Items commonly sucked such as metal hair clips, pencils (cobalt paint or metals), etc;
- Essential oils;
- Wooden and nickel mouthpieces of musical instruments.

Clinical features

There may be persistent irritation and scaling of the vermilion or a more acute reaction with oedema and vesiculation (Figure 7.11).

Diagnosis

The diagnosis is clinical; erythema multiforme may present similarly but usually also with oral or other erosions. If an allergic reaction is

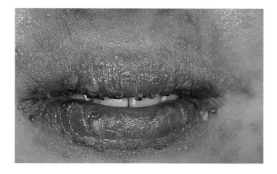

Figure 7.11
Contact cheilitis

suspected, patch tests should be carried out using the appropriate concentrations of the substances concerned.

Management

- The offending substance should be traced and avoided;
- Topical corticosteroids often give symptomatic relief.

Double lip

Double lip is a developmental anomaly usually involving the upper lip. A fold of redundant tissue is found on the inner aspect of the involved lip. Double lip may occur alone or in association with other anomalies. The association with blepharochalasis (laxity of the upper eyelid skin) and sometimes nontoxic thyroid enlargement is known as Ascher's syndrome. Double lip requires no treatment except for cosmetic purposes.

Erythema multiforme

Definition

Erythema multiforme is an often recurrent disorder affecting mucocutaneous tissues, and characterized by serosanguinous exudates on the lips, and sometimes target-like lesions on skin.

Incidence

Uncommon

Age mainly affected

Younger adults

Sex mainly affected

M>F

Aetiology

Erythema multiforme (EM) appears to be an immunologically related reaction with sub- and intraepithelial vesiculation, the aetiology of which includes:

- Infections (such as herpes simplex or mycoplasma);
- Drugs (sulphonamides, cephalosporins, barbiturates, hydantoins, cimetidine and others); this form is increasingly termed toxic epidermal necrolysis;
- Food additives such as benzoates;
- A range of other trigger factors (Figures 7.12 and 7.13).

Minor EM appears related mainly to herpes simplex; major EM is precipitated mainly by drugs or mycoplasma.

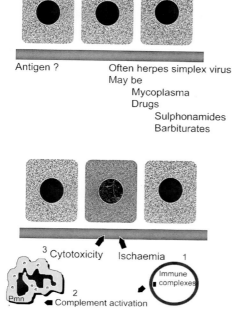

Figure 7.12
Erythema multiforme;
aetiopathogenesis

Figure 7.13
Erythema multiforme;
aetiopathogenesis (Pmn
– polymorphonuclear
leukocytes)

Clinical features

Usually attacks last for 10–14 days once or twice a year. The oral lesions often recur, but the condition usually resolves after 6 or 7 episodes within a mean period of 3 years (range 10–25 years). The periodicity can vary from weeks to years.

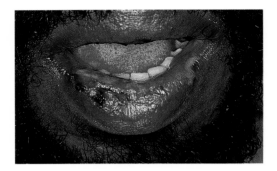

Figure 7.14
*Erythema multiforme;
typical labial swelling,
ulceration and scabbing.*

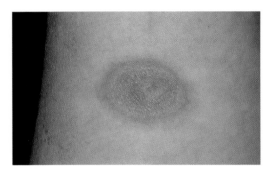

Figure 7.15
*Erythema multiforme;
target (iris) lesion on skin*

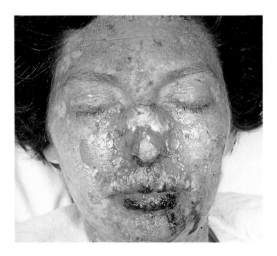

Figure 7.16
*Stevens–Johnson
syndrome: major
erythema multiforme
affecting mouth, other
mucosa and skin*

- The minor form affects only one site. Erythema multiforme may affect mouth alone, or skin and/or other mucosae (Figure 7.14). Rashes are various but typically 'iris' or 'target' lesions or bullae on extremities (Figure 7.15);

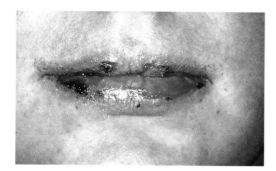

Figure 7.17
*Erythema multiforme:
blood-stained crusting of
lips*

- The major form (Stevens–Johnson syndrome) causes widespread lesions affecting mouth, eyes, pharynx, larynx, oesophagus, skin and genitals, with fever and toxicity, bullous and other rashes, pneumonia, arthritis, nephritis or myocarditis (Figure 7.16).

Oral lesions include:

- Lips: cracked, bleeding, crusted, swollen (Figure 7.17);
- Ulcers: diffuse and widespread (Figures 7.18–7.21).

Oral lesions progress through macules to blisters and ulceration, typically most pronounced in the anterior parts of the mouth. Extensive oral ulceration may be seen.

Other lesions in some patients include:

- Rash: typically target, or iris-like, but may be bullous (Figure 7.22);
- Ocular changes that resemble those of mucous membrane pemphigoid: dry eyes and symblepharon may result;
- Balanitis, urethritis and vulval ulcers.

Diagnosis

- The diagnosis is mainly clinical;
- Virological studies may be indicated if differentiation from acute herpetic stomatitis is difficult;
- Biopsy may be indicated but is not always helpful. There may be sub- or intraepithelial vesiculation, but pathology can be variable and immunostaining is not specific. Immunostaining shows fibrin and C3 at the epithelial basement membrane zone, and perivascular IgM, C3 and fibrin.

Management

- Precipitating factors, when identified, should be treated;

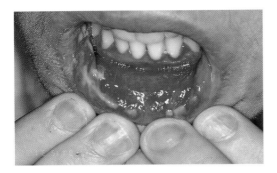

Figure 7.18
*Erythema multiforme:
ulceration mainly in the
anterior mouth*

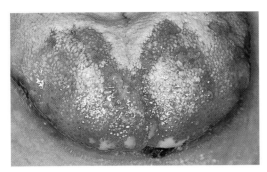

Figure 7.19
Erythema multiforme

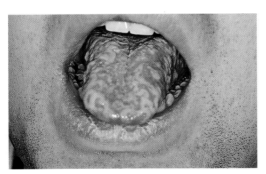

Figure 7.20
*Erythema multiforme:
widespread ulceration*

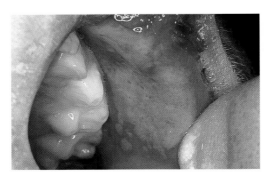

Figure 7.21
*Erythema multiforme:
extensive ulceration*

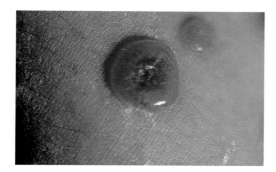

Figure 7.22
Erythema multiforme; bullous rash

- No specific treatment is available;
- Aciclovir may be indicated in EM related to herpes simplex virus;
- Oral hygiene should be improved with 0.2% aqueous chlorhexidine mouthbaths.

In addition:

- Minor EM not responding to symptomatic treatment may require systemic corticosteroids;
- Major EM should be treated with systemic corticosteroids and/or azathioprine or other immunomodulatory drugs. Levamisole and thalidomide have occasionally been used to some effect;
- Patients with major forms such as the Stevens–Johnson syndrome may need to be admitted for hospital care.

Exfoliative cheilitis (factitious cheilitis)

Definition

Exfoliative cheilitis is a chronic superficial inflammatory disorder of the vermilion of the lips characterized by persistent scaling.

Incidence

Rare

Age mainly affected

Adolescents and young adults

Sex mainly affected

F>M

Aetiology

- Thought often to be factitious, owing to repeated lip sucking, chewing or other manipulation of the lips;
- The majority of patients have a personality disorder;
- The patient can sometimes be observed frequently biting or sucking the lips;
- In some cases the condition appears to start with chapping or with atopic eczema, and develops into a habit tic.

Clinical features

The process, which often starts in the middle of the lower lip and spreads to involve the whole of the lower or both lips, consists of scaling and crusting of the vermilion persisting in varying severity for months or years. Chronic exfoliative cheilitis is readily contaminated by candida. In such cases the clinical features are variable and may simulate carcinoma, lichen planus or lupus erythematosus.

Diagnosis

The diagnosis is now restricted to those few patients whose lesions cannot be attributed to other causes such as contact sensitization or light (see actinic cheilitis, page 306).

Management

- Contact and actinic cheilitis must be carefully excluded;
- Some cases resolve spontaneously;
- Reassurance and topical corticosteroids may be helpful;
- Others require psychotherapy or tranquillizers.

Granulomatous cheilitis (Miescher's cheilitis)

Definition

A chronic swelling of the lip due to granulomatous inflammation of unknown cause

Incidence

Rare

Age mainly affected

Adolescents and young adults

Sex mainly affected

F>M

Aetiology

The cause is unknown. Biopsy of the tissues during the early stages of the disease shows only oedema and perivascular lymphocytic infiltration. In some cases of long duration no other changes are seen, but in others the infiltrate becomes more dense and pleomorphic and small focal granulomas are formed, indistinguishable from sarcoidosis, OFG or Crohn's disease. Some cases may represent a localized form of sarcoidosis or ectopic Crohn's disease or orofacial granulomatosis. A few patients react to cobalt or to food additives such as cinnamic aldehyde, though these reactions are by no means always relevant.

Clinical features

The essential feature of the syndrome is granulomatous swelling of lip or face. The earliest manifestation is sudden diffuse or nodular swellings involving the upper lip, the lower lip and one or both cheeks. In the first episode the oedema typically subsides completely in hours or days, but after recurrent attacks the swelling may persist, and slowly increases in degree (Figure 7.23). It gradually becomes firmer and eventually acquires the consistency of firm rubber. After some years, the swelling may very slowly regress.

Miescher's cheilitis: in this, the granulomatous changes are confined to the lip; this is generally regarded as a monosymptomatic form

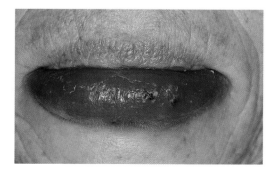

Figure 7.23
Granulomatous cheilitis

of the Melkersson–Rosenthal syndrome, although the possibility remains that these may be two separate diseases.

Melkersson–Rosenthal syndrome: in this, labial oedema is seen in association with recurrent facial palsy and added scrotal tongue. A fissured or scrotal tongue is present from birth in some, which may indicate genetic susceptibility. Facial palsy is of the lower motor-neurone type. It may precede the attacks of oedema by months or years, but more commonly develops later.

Diagnosis

In the early attacks, clinical differentiation from angioedema may be impossible in the absence of either scrotal tongue or facial palsy. Persistence of the swelling between attacks should suggest the diagnosis, which can sometimes be confirmed by biopsy. However, the histological changes are not always conspicuous or specific. In the established cases, other causes of macrocheilia (see Table 7.3) must be excluded. Ascher's syndrome associated with blepharochalasia is likely to cause confusion, although the swelling of the lip is caused by redundant salivary tissue and is present from childhood (page 320).

Management

- Reactions to dietary components should be sought and possible antigens avoided;
- The injection of triamcinolone into the lips after local analgesia may be effective;
- Clofazimine appears to help many patients;
- Systemic corticosteroids are rarely indicated.

Herpes labialis

Herpes is discussed in Chapter 4, and therefore a synopsis only is given here.

Definition

Recurrent blistering of the lips caused by reactivation of herpes simplex virus (HSV).

Incidence

Up to 15% of the population have recurrent HSV infections.

Age mainly affected

Adults

Sex mainly affected

M=F

Aetiology

HSV is latent in the trigeminal ganglion. Factors such as fever, sunlight, trauma or immunosuppression can reactivate the virus which is shed into saliva, and there may be clinical recrudescence, recurrently, to produce herpes labialis.

Clinical features

Lesions are typically at the mucocutaneous junction. They start as macules that rapidly become papular, vesicular and then pustular. They scab and heal usually without scarring (Figure 7.24 and Chapter 4). Widespread recalcitrant lesions may appear in immunocompromised patients (Figure 7.25).

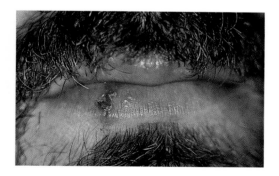

Figure 7.24
Recurrent herpes labialis

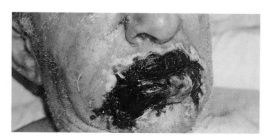

Figure 7.25
Recurrent herpes labialis in immunocompromised patient

Diagnosis

Diagnosis is largely clinical though viral culture, immunodetection or electron microscopy are used very occasionally. Assay of serum antibodies gives little help.

Management

- Penciclovir 1% cream or possibly aciclovir 5% cream applied in the prodrome may help abort or control lesions in healthy patients (Table 10.9);
- Systemic aciclovir or other antivirals may be needed for immunocompromised patients.

Kawasaki disease

See Mucocutaneous lymph node syndrome (page 334)

Labial melanotic macule (solitary labial lentigo)

Definition

Small brown macule

Incidence

Common

Age mainly affected

Adult

Sex mainly affected

F>M

Aetiology

Physiological or reactive

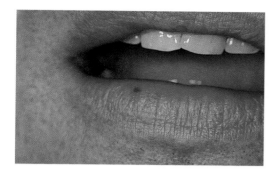

Figure 7.26
Melanotic macule

Clinical features

Usually a solitary, very small, asymptomatic brown macule unchanging in character (Figure 7.26). They may resemble ephelides, although these tend to fade in winter and darken in summer. Most are near the midline, on the lower lip vermilion. Occasionally they grow rapidly or are multiple or large.

Diagnosis

Clinically, the labial melanotic macule may resemble early melanoma if it develops rapidly and then should be excised for histopathological examination. Histopathologically, the lip or mucosal epithelium is normal apart from increased pigmentation of the basal layer, accentuated at the tips of rete ridges.

Management

- Excise for diagnostic or cosmetic reasons; or
- Hide by lipstick.

Lip fissure

A fissure may develop in the lip where there is a hereditary predisposition for weakness in the first branchial arch fusion and in:

- Mouth breathing (Figure 7.27);
- Exposure to sun, wind, cold weather and smoking;
- Down's syndrome;
- Oral Crohn's disease;

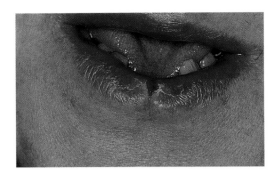

Figure 7.27
Lip fissure

- Orofacial granulomatosis;
- Atopic dermatitis.

Lip fissures are fortunately uncommon. Contrary to the clinical impression that fissures are seen mainly in the lower lip there is a higher prevalence in the upper lip. The fissure typically is:

- Median or paramedian and runs from the oral side of the vermilion across towards the skin but is usually restricted to the lip;
- Painful;
- Likely to bleed;
- Liable to infection with *Staphylococcus aureus*.

Management

- Local applications of bland creams (e.g. E45, Boots, Nottingham) should be tried first;
- If that fails, antimicrobials should be tried;
- Corticosteroids, silver nitrate or salicylic acid may be effective;
- Excision, preferably with a Z-plasty may finally be needed.

Lip pit and fistula

Definition

Lip pits are blind epithelial-lined developmental anomalies paramedial or at the commissures.

Incidence

Uncommon

Age mainly affected

From birth

Sex mainly affected

M=F

Aetiology

Genetic; often autosomal dominant

Clinical features

Commissural pits are:

- Unilateral or bilateral;
- Distinct definite pits ranging from 1 to 4 mm in diameter and depth (Figure 7.28);
- Present from infancy;
- Sometimes associated with aural sinuses or pits;
- Rarely may be infected and present as recurrent or refractory angular cheilitis.

Paramedian pits:

- Are usually on the lower lip;
- Are usually bilateral and symmetrical often just to one side of the philtrum;
- May exude mucus;
- Are often associated with cleft lip or palate.

Lip fistulae:

- May be isolated;

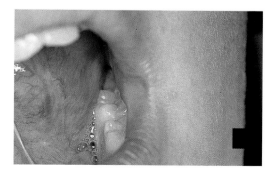

Figure 7.28
Lip pit (commissural pit)

- May be associated with clefts, or the Van der Woude syndrome, orofacial digital syndrome 1 or popliteal pterygium.

Diagnosis

Clinical

Management

Surgically remove for cosmetic purposes if necessary.

Lip ulcer due to calibre-persistent artery

A 'calibre-persistent artery' is defined as an artery with a diameter larger than normal near a mucosal or external surface. The ulcer is attributed to continual pulsation from the large artery running parallel to the surface, though the exact mechanism is obscure. Ligation of the artery appears successful.

Mucocutaneous lymph node syndrome (Kawasaki disease)

Definition

An idiopathic childhood disease manifesting with rash, desquamation, cheilitis and sometimes myocarditis

Incidence

Rare

Age mainly affected

Childhood

Sex mainly affected

M=F

Aetiology

Idiopathic but apparently of infectious aetiology

Clinical features

- Generalized lymphadenopathy;
- A rash with desquamation of hands and feet;
- Oedematous lips and cheilitis;
- Pharyngitis;
- Myocarditis in a minority.

Diagnosis

There is no specific diagnostic test.

Management

There is no specific treatment.

Plasma cell cheilitis

Definition

Plasma cell cheilitis is characterized by dense plasma cell infiltrates in the lips and other mucosae close to body orifices.

Incidence

Rare

Age mainly affected

Elderly

Sex mainly affected

M=F

Aetiology

An idiopathic benign inflammatory condition

Clinical features

Circumscribed flat or elevated erythematous patches usually on the lower lip

Diagnosis

Clinical and biopsy

Management

- Potent topical corticosteroids such as clobetasol, or
- Triamcinolone injection.

Venous lake (venous varix, senile haemangioma of lip)

Definition

Dilated venous space lined by a single layer of flattened endothelial cells with a thick wall of fibrous tissue.

Incidence

Uncommon

Age mainly affected

Middle-aged and elderly

Sex mainly affected

M=F

Aetiology

Idiopathic

Clinical features

This is a bluish-purple soft swelling, 2–10 mm in diameter, usually on the lower lip. The lesion empties on prolonged pressure.

Diagnosis

Clinical

Management

A venous lake may be only a trivial cosmetic problem or it can bleed severely after trauma. It can be excised, but careful cryotherapy, electrocautery or treatment with the argon laser can also give good results.

Further reading

Brook IM, King DJ, Miller ID. Chronic granulomatous cheilitis and its relationship to Crohn's disease. *Oral Surg Oral Med Oral Pathol* (1983) **56**: 405–7.

Brooke RL. Exfoliative cheilitis. *Oral Surg Oral Med Oral Pathol* (1978) **45**: 52–55.

Buchner A, Hansen LS. Pigmented nevi of the oral mucosa. *Oral Surg Oral Med Oral Pathol* (1980) **49**: 55–62.

Burton J, Scully C. The lips. In: Champion RH, Burton J, Burns DA, Breathnach SM, eds, *Textbook of Dermatology*, 6th edn. (Blackwells: Oxford, 1998) 3124.

Chandler K, Chaudhry Z, Kumar N et al. Melanocanthoma: a rare cause of oral hyperpigmentation. *Oral Surg Oral Med Oral Pathol Oral Radiol Endod* (1997) **84**: 492–4.

Eveson JW, Scully C. *Colour Atlas of Oral Pathology*. (London, Mosby-Wolfe: 1995).

Fisher AA. Allergic contact dermatitis from musical instruments. *Cutis* (1993) **51**: 75–6.

Ho KKL, Dervan P, O'Loughlin S et al. Labial melanotic macule: a clinical histopathologic and ultrastructural study. *J Am Acad Dermatol* (1993) **28**: 33–9.

Jones JH, Mason DK. *Oral Manifestations of Systemic Disease*, 2nd edn. (Baillière: London, 1980).

Kaugars GE, Heise AP, Riley WT et al. Oral melanotic macules. A review of 353 cases. *Oral Surg Oral Med Oral Pathol* (1993) **76**: 59–61.

Millard HD, Mason DK, eds. *Perspectives on 1993 World Workshop on Oral Medicine*. (University of Michigan Press: Ann Arbor, 1998).

Ohman SC, Dahlen G, Moller A, Ohman A. Angular cheilitis: a clinical and microbial study. *J Oral Pathol* (1986) **15**: 213–17.

Page LR, Corio RL, Crawford BE. The oral melanotic macule. *Oral Surg Oral Med Oral Pathol* (1977) **44**: 219–26.

Reade PC, Sim R. Exfoliative cheilitis: a factitious disorder? *Int J Oral Maxillofac Surg* (1986) **15**: 313–17.

Reinish EI, Raviv M, Srolovitz H et al. Tongue, primary amyloidosis and multiple myeloma. *Oral Surg Oral Med Oral Pathol* (1994) **77**: 121–5.

Rodu B, Martinez MG. Peutz–Jeghers syndrome and cancer. *Oral Surg Oral Med Oral Pathol* (1984) **58**: 584–8.

Scully C. Diagnosis and diagnostic procedures: general and soft tissue diagnosis. In: *Pathways in Practice.* (Faculty of General Dental Practice, Royal College of Surgeons of England 1993) 25–33.

Scully C. The pathology of orofacial disease. In: Barnes IE, Walls AWG, eds, *Gerodontology.* (Wright-Butterworths: Oxford, 1994) 29–41.

Scully C. Prevention of oral mucosal disease. In: Murray JJ, ed., *Prevention of Oral and Dental Disease,* 3rd edn. (Oxford University Press: Oxford, 1995) 160–72.

Scully C. The oral cavity. In: Champion RH, Burton J, Burns DA, Breathnach SM, eds, *Textbook of Dermatology,* 6th edn. (Blackwells: Oxford, 1998) 3047–123.

Scully C. The oral cavity. In: Champion RH, Burton J, Ebling FJG, eds, *Textbook of Dermatology,* 6th edn. (Blackwells: Oxford, 1998).

Scully C, Cawson RA. *Medical Problems in Dentistry,* 4th edn. (Butterworth-Heinemann: Oxford, 1998).

Scully C, Porter SR. Oral mucosal disease: a decade of new entities, aetiologies and associations. *Int Dental J* (1994) **44**: 33–43.

Scully C, Welbury R. *Colour Atlas of Oral Disease in Children and Adolescents.* (Mosby-Wolfe: London, 1994).

Scully C, Flint S, Porter S. *Oral Diseases.* (Martin Dunitz: London, 1996).

Scully C, Bagan J, Eisen D et al. *Dermatology of the Lips.* (Isis: Oxford, 2000).

Swerlick RA, Cooper PH. Cheilitis glandularis: a re-evaluation. *J Am Acad Dermatol* (1984) **10**: 466–72.

van der Waal N, van der Kwast WA, van der Waal I. Median rhomboid glossitis: a follow-up of 16 patients. *J Oral Med* (1986) **41**: 117–20.

Winchester L, Scully C, Prime SS et al. Cheilitis glandularis: a case affecting the upper lip. *Oral Surg Oral Med Oral Pathol* (1986) **62**: 654–7.

8

Palate complaints

Surprisingly few mucosal conditions affect the palate.

Blisters

Blisters are uncommon except in:

- Burns;
- Pemphigoid;
- Superficial mucoceles;
- Angina bullosa haemorrhagica.

Lumps

Unerupted teeth and tori (Figure 8.24) are the most common congenital causes of lumps in the palate. Acquired conditions causing swellings include:

- Dental abscess pointing on the palate (usually from the palatal roots of the first and second maxillary molars, or from upper lateral incisors) (Figure 8.1);
- Cysts;
- Fibrous lumps;
- Papillomas;
- Carcinoma;
- Kaposi's sarcoma;
- Lymphomas;
- Pleomorphic adenomas and other salivary neoplasms (Chapter 5 and Figures 8.2 and 8.3);
- Adenomatoid hyperplasia;
- Necrotizing sialometaplasia;
- Invasive carcinoma from the maxillary sinus;

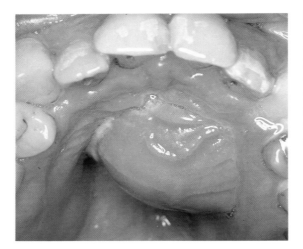

Figure 8.1
Dental abscess: most abscesses cause a buccal swelling but those arising on a maxillary lateral incisor or first molar may cause palatal swelling

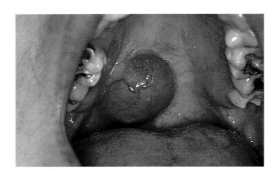

Figure 8.2
Pleomorphic salivary adenoma

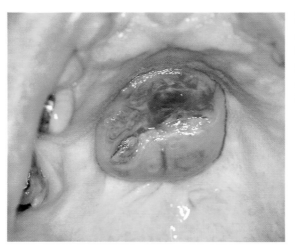

Figure 8.3
Salivary neoplasm arising from minor glands in the soft palate/hard palate junction

- Fibrous dysplasia;
- Paget's disease.

Red lesions

Red lesions may be caused by:

- Erythematous candidiasis (Figures 8.4 and 8.5), mainly denture-induced stomatitis, the most common cause of redness in the palate;
- Burns;
- Petechiae and ecchymoses (Figure 8.6);
- Pemphigus;
- Angina bullosa haemorrhagica;
- Mucositis;
- Erythroplasia;

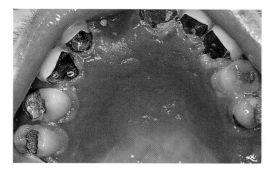

Figure 8.4
Chronic erythematous candidiasis

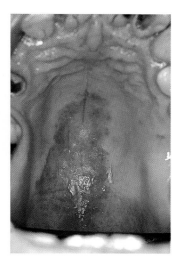

Figure 8.5
*Erythematous candidiasis
in HIV disease
producing an
erythematous fingerprint
lesion*

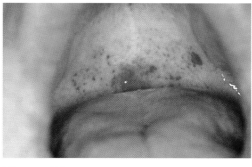

Figure 8.6
Petechiae

- Lupus erythematosus;
- Reiter's syndrome;
- Graft-versus-host disease;
- Telangiectasia;
- Angiomas;
- Kaposi's sarcoma.

Ulceration

Ulcers are uncommon in the hard palate except in:

- Infections (herpetic stomatitis: Figure 8.7, Coxsackie virus infections: Figure 8.8, syphilis, deep mycoses), skin diseases (pemphigus: Figure 8.9, pemphigoid, lupus erythematosus);
- Neoplasms;
- Pyostomatitis vegetans.

Ulcers of the fauces may be seen particularly in:

- Aphthous stomatitis;
- Herpes simplex or Coxsackie virus infection;
- Lymphomas.

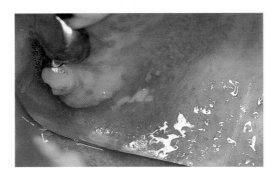

Figure 8.7
Herpes simplex recurrence in a typical site which often follows a local analgesic injection over the greater palatine foramen

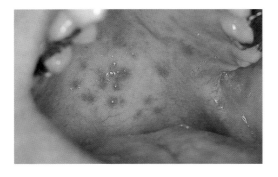

Figure 8.8
Herpangina: typically a Coxsackie virus infection

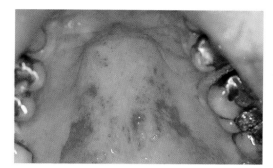

Figure 8.9
Pemphigus vulgaris

White lesions

White lesions in the palate may be seen in:

- Smoker's keratosis (Figure 8.10);
- Candidiasis (Figure 8.11);
- Lupus erythematosus;
- Lichen planus;

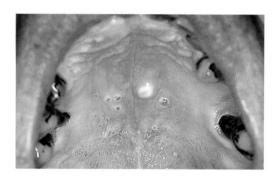

Figure 8.10
Smoker's keratosis

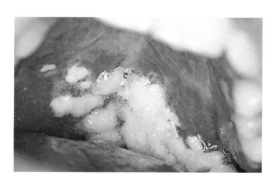

Figure 8.11
Thrush in a leukaemic patient

- Various congenital disorders;
- Verruciform xanthoma is a rare cause;
- Darier's disease is a rare cause.

Adenomatoid hyperplasia

Adenomatoid hyperplasia is a benign swelling typically of minor salivary glands in the palate. Of unknown aetiology, possibly related to irritation by smoking or a denture, the condition is self-limiting.

Angina bullosa haemorrhagica (localized oral purpura)

Definition

Spontaneously appearing blood blisters in patients with no haemostatic defect

Incidence

Uncommon

Age mainly affected

Elderly

Sex mainly affected

M=F

Aetiology

- Unclear, though minor trauma appears to provoke the blistering;
- This is a disorder affecting older persons, perhaps analogous to senile purpura;
- No bleeding tendency appears to underlie this condition;
- No autoimmunity appears to underlie this condition;
- Corticosteroid inhalers may sometimes predispose.

Clinical features

- Blood blisters are seen in the mouth or pharynx, mainly on the soft palate (Figure 8.12) and occasionally on the lateral border of the tongue or buccal mucosa (Figure 8.13);
- Blisters are typically solitary, large and confined to one side of the soft palate (Figure 8.14);
- There is rapid onset of blistering over minutes, with breakdown in a day or two to a large round ulcer that heals spontaneously (Figure 8.15).

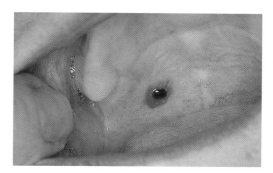

Figure 8.12
Angina bullosa haemorrhagica

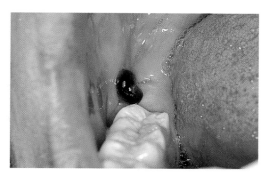

Figure 8.13
Angina bullosa haemorrhagica

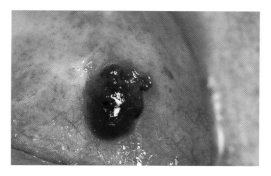

Figure 8.14
Angina bullosa haemorrhagica: a typical unilateral blood-filled blister

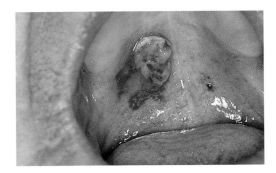

Figure 8.15
Angina bullosa haemorrhagica: collapsed blister

Diagnosis

It is necessary to differentiate this from pemphigoid and other vesiculobullous disorders, trauma, amyloidosis and purpura. Confirm haemostasis is normal first and biopsy to exclude pemphigoid, if that is likely.

Management

- There is no specific treatment other than reassurance;
- It may be helpful to burst the blister;
- Topical analgesics may provide symptomatic relief.

Denture-induced stomatitis (denture sore mouth; chronic atrophic candidiasis)

Definition

Diffuse erythema limited to denture-bearing area

Incidence

Common

Age mainly affected

Middle aged and elderly

Sex mainly affected

F>M

Aetiology

This condition is found exclusively in people who wear appliances (dentures or orthodontic plates). Trauma is an unlikely cause, since there is less trauma beneath an upper than a lower appliance and virtually all cases affect the palate.

It usually:

- Is seen only under an upper appliance;
- Affects only the mucosa in contact with the denture fitting surface, a fact that makes it quite clear that it is not caused by an allergic reaction, which would affect any mucosa in contact with the appliance;
- Appears to be related to the proliferation of microorganisms (*Candida albicans* mainly but occasionally *Streptococcus milleri* and klebsiella) beneath and within the appliance-fitting surface.

Clinical features

- Usually asymptomatic;
- May be an associated angular stomatitis;
- Diffuse erythema limited to denture-bearing area and classified (Newton) into three types: Punctate erythema (Figure 8.16); Uniform erythema (Figure 8.17); and Hyperplastic (see Papillary hyperplasia) (Figure 8.18).

Management

- Improve denture hygiene;
- Keep dentures out of the mouth at night; clean and store in 1% hypochlorite or 0.2% aqueous chlorhexidine;

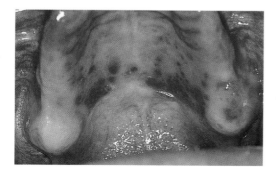

Figure 8.16
Chronic atrophic candidiasis: Newton type 1

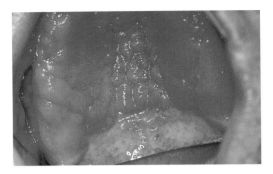

Figure 8.17
Chronic atrophic candidiasis:
Newton type 2

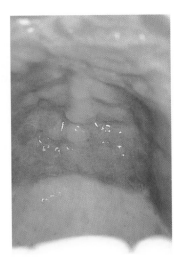

Figure 8.18
Chronic atrophic
candidiasis: Newton type 3

- Antifungals (mainly required where there is also angular stomatitis) (Table 10.8);
- Attention to dentures.

Kaposi's sarcoma

Definition

An endothelial proliferative condition widely regarded as a neoplasm

Incidence

Uncommon

Age mainly affected

Mainly 2nd to 4th decades

Sex mainly affected

M>F

Aetiology

Kaposi's sarcoma (KS) is a malignant endothelial tumour probably induced by a recently described virus: human herpesvirus 8. It is seen almost exclusively in AIDS, or other immunocompromised patients. Rarely, it is seen in elderly Jews and those of Mediterranean or Middle Eastern origin, in the absence of an identified immune defect.

Clinical features

Kaposi's sarcoma typically:

- Produces a red, bluish or purple, sometimes brown, macule (Figure 8.19), which then increases to a nodule and may ulcerate (Figure 8.20);
- Is seen primarily in the skin and mucosa in the head and neck, especially on the nose;
- Is seen in the palate, over the greater palatine vessels or the anterior maxillary labial gingivae;
- Is part of much more widespread disease.

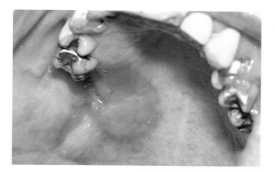

Figure 8.19
Kaposi's sarcoma: an early dusky brown or purple macule in a typical site

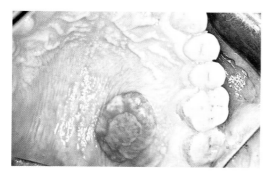

Figure 8.20
Kaposi's sarcoma: nodular stage

Diagnosis

- Biopsy is confirmatory;
- An HIV test may be indicated after appropriate counselling.

Diagnosis is often fairly obvious but it may be necessary to differentiate from other pigmented lesions, especially haemangiomas, purpura, or epithelioid angiomatosis (a bacterial infection with *Rochalimaea Bartonella henseleae*, that responds to antibiotics).

Management

The underlying predisposing condition should be treated if possible. Oral lesions respond to radiotherapy or to vinca alkaloids systemically or intralesionally.

Malignant melanoma

Definition

Melanoma is a rare malignant neoplasm of melanocytes, with a poor prognosis.

Incidence

Rare

Age mainly affected

Middle-aged

Sex mainly affected

M=F

Aetiology

Extraoral melanoma is increasing in frequency as a result of increased sun exposure.

Clinical features

Malignant melanoma may arise in apparently normal mucosa or in a pre-existent pigmented naevus, usually in the palate, occasionally the upper alveolus or gingiva (Figure 4.140). Features suggestive of malignancy include:

- Rapid increase in size;
- Change in colour;
- Ulceration;
- Pain;
- Occurrence of satellite pigmented spots;
- Regional lymph node enlargement.

Diagnosis

The consensus of opinion is that lesions suspected of being malignant melanomas should not be biopsied until the time of definitive operation, but the prognosis is poor unless treatment is exceptionally early.

Malignant melanoma is classified with increasingly poor prognosis into:

- Lentigo maligna;
- Superficial spreading melanoma;
- Nodular melanoma.

Management

Surgery

Papillary hyperplasia

The vault of the hard palate may occasionally show small multiple nodules about 2 mm in diameter, termed papillary hyperplasia. Causes include:

- Denture-induced stomatitis usually (Figure 8.18);
- Poor oral hygiene;
- HIV infection rarely;
- Drugs capable of producing gingival hyperplasia rarely.

The underlying cause should be sought and treated. Residual hyperplasia may be excised surgically with scalpel, electrosurgery or laser.

Stomatitis nicotina (smoker's palate; smoker's keratosis; nicotinic stomatitis; stomatitis palatini; leukokeratosis nicotina palati)

Definition

This is a diffuse white lesion covering most of the hard palate, related to tobacco smoking.

Incidence

Uncommon

Age mainly affected

Middle-aged or elderly adults

Sex mainly affected

M>F

Aetiology

Smoker's keratosis is seen among heavy, long-term pipe smokers and some cigar smokers, and only occasionally with the far more common habit of cigarette smoking, but it can be seen in heavy smokers. Similar lesions have rarely been seen in persons using reverse smoking, menthol lozenges or taking very hot drinks.

Clinical features

The appearance of smoker's keratosis is distinctive (Figure 8.10) in that the following occur:

- The palate is affected;
- Any part protected by a denture is spared (Figure 8.21);
- The lesion has two components, namely hyperkeratosis and inflammatory swelling of minor mucous glands leading to white thickening of the palatal mucosa in a polygonal cobblestoned fashion (Figures 8.21 and 8.22) associated with small umbilicated swellings with red centres;

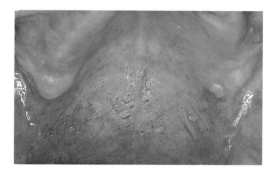

Figure 8.21
*Smoker's keratosis seen
mainly in the soft palate
which was unprotected
by a denture*

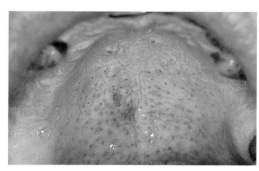

Figure 8.22
Smoker's keratosis

• The maxillary teeth in particular are heavily stained from the tobacco use.

Diagnosis and management

The clinical appearances and history are so distinctive that biopsy should not normally be necessary. The patient should be encouraged to stop the causative habit.

Torus palatinus

Definition

This is a developmental benign exostosis in the palate.

Incidence

Common; seen especially in Asians, Mongoloids and Inuits.

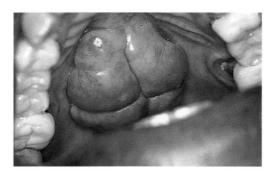

Figure 8.23
Torus palatinus: a rather extreme example

Age mainly affected

Seen mainly after puberty

Sex mainly affected

F>M

Aetiology

Developmental exostosis

Clinical features

- Seen in the centre of the hard palate (Figures 8.23 and 8.24);
- Overlying mucosa is normal and typically of normal colour;
- Painless;
- Bony hard smooth or nodular surface.

Diagnosis

Clinical

Management

Tori are typically of no consequence, apart from occasionally interfering with denture construction. They should usually be left alone.

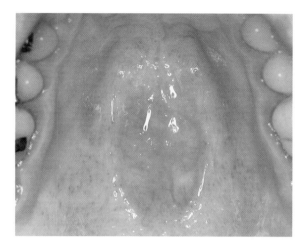

Figure 8.24
Torus palatinus

Further reading

Scully C. The oral cavity. In: Champion RH, Burton J, Ebling FJG, eds, *Textbook of Dermatology*, 5th edn (Blackwells: Oxford, 1991) 2689–769.

Scully C. Diagnosis and diagnostic procedures: general and soft tissue diagnosis. In: *Pathways in Practice* (Faculty of General Dental Practice, Royal College of Surgeons of England, 1993) 25–33.

Scully C. Prevention of oral mucosal disease. In: Murray JJ, ed., *Prevention of Oral and Dental Disease*, 3rd edn. (Oxford University Press: Oxford, 1994) 160–72.

Scully C. The pathology of orofacial disease. In: Barnes IE, Walls AWG, eds, *Gerodontology*. (Wright-Butterworths: Oxford, 1994) 29–41.

Scully C. The oral cavity. In: Champion RH, Burton J, Burns DA, Breathnach SM, eds, *Textbook of Dermatology*, 6th edn. (Blackwells: Oxford, 1998).

Scully C, Cawson RA. *Medical Problems in Dentistry*, 4th edn. (Butterworth-Heinemann: Oxford, 1998).

Scully C, Porter SR. Oral mucosal disease: a decade of new entities, aetiologies and associations. *Int Dent J* (1994) **44**: 33–43.

Scully C, Welbury R. *Colour Atlas of Oral Disease in Children and Adolescents*. (Mosby-Wolfe: London, 1994).

Scully C, Flint S, Porter S. *Oral Diseases*. (Martin Dunitz: London, 1996).

9

Tongue complaints

The tongue is divided by a V-shaped groove, the sulcus terminalis, into an anterior two-thirds and a posterior third. Various papillae on the dorsum include the filiform papillae, which cover the entire anterior surface and form an abrasive surface to control the food bolus as it is pressed against the palate, and the fungiform papillae. The latter are mushroom-shaped, red structures covered by nonkeratinized epithelium. They are scattered between the filiform papillae and have taste buds on their surface. Adjacent and anterior to the sulcus terminalis are 8–12 large circumvallate papillae, each surrounded by a deep groove into which open the ducts of serous minor salivary glands. The lateral walls of these papillae contain taste buds. The foliate papillae consist of 4–11 parallel ridges, alternating with deep grooves in the mucosa, on the lateral margins on the posterior part of the tongue. There are taste buds on their lateral walls.

Taste from the anterior two-thirds of the tongue is mediated via the chorda tympani nerve and runs with the facial nerve. The glossopharyngeal nerve carries taste sensation from the posterior tongue.

The lingual tonsils are found on the posterior dorsum of the tongue as oval prominences with intervening lingual crypts lined by nonkeratinized epithelium. They are part of Waldeyer's oropharyngeal ring of lymphoid tissue.

Beneath the tongue is seen the frenulum and folds running posteriorly, termed plicae fimbriatae.

Amyloidosis

Definition

Amyloidosis is a rare condition characterized by deposition in tissues of an eosinophilic hyaline material, amyloid, which has a fibrillar structure on electron microscopy.

Incidence

Rare

Age mainly affected

Middle-aged and elderly

Sex mainly affected

M=F

Aetiology

Amyloid deposits

- In primary (including myeloma-associated) amyloid, deposits consist of immunoglobulin light chains;
- In secondary and other forms of amyloid (now seen mainly in rheumatoid arthritis and ulcerative colitis) consist of AA proteins.

Clinical features

Oral amyloidosis is seen almost exclusively in primary amyloidosis. Manifestations include:

- Macroglossia, in up to 50% of patients; this is a poor prognostic finding (Figure 9.1);

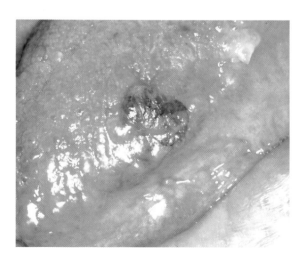

Figure 9.1
Amyloidosis producing macroglossia and petechiae

- Oral petechiae or blood-filled bullae.

Diagnosis

Investigations are required to confirm the diagnosis and to exclude myelomatosis, and may include the following:

- Lesional biopsy: oral deposits may be detected histologically even in absence of clinically apparent lesions. Congo red or thioflavine T staining of a biopsy usually confirm the diagnosis, though, in extreme cases, the deposits are seen on conventional haematoxylin and eosin staining. Note the patients may have a bleeding tendency;
- Labial salivary gland biopsy: may be positive even in the absence of clinical oral lesions;
- Blood picture and erythrocyte sedimentation rate;
- Urinalysis (Bence–Jones proteinuria) for myeloma;
- Serum and urine electrophoresis for myeloma;
- Skeletal survey for myeloma;
- Bone marrow biopsy for myeloma.

Management

- Management is of the underlying disease. Chemotherapy with melphalan, corticosteroids or fluoxymesterone are usually used;
- Surgical reduction of the tongue is inadvisable since the tissue is friable, often bleeds excessively and the swelling quickly recurs.

Ankyloglossia (tongue tie)

Definition

Tongue tie: a tight lingual frenulum

Incidence

Up to 1.7%

Age mainly affected

From birth

Sex mainly affected

M=F

Aetiology

Genetic in most cases. There are occasional associations with:

- Cocaine-addicted mothers;
- Trisomy 13;
- Pierre–Robin syndrome.

Scleroderma or other causes of scarring such as after hemi-glossecto-my may rarely produce acquired ankyloglossia.

Clinical features

- The frenulum is short (Figure 9.2);
- Ankyloglossia is usually of little consequence, though it may impair breast feeding, and does not interfere with speech;
- The main consequence of ankyloglossia can be difficulty in using the tongue to cleanse food away from the teeth and vestibules.

Diagnosis

Clinical

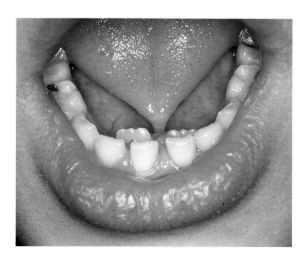

Figure 9.2
Ankyloglossia (tongue tie). The double row of incisors is unrelated and simply caused by permanent incisors erupting while the deciduous incisors remain to be exfoliated

Management

Surgery if there are real complications

Black hairy tongue

Definition

Black hairy tongue affects the dorsum of the tongue; the filiform papillae are excessively long and stained.

Incidence

Uncommon

Age mainly affected

Elderly

Sex mainly affected

M>F

Aetiology

Black hairy tongue is more likely to be seen in those who are:

* Edentulous;
* On a soft, nonabrasive diet;
* Poor at oral hygiene;
* Smokers;
* Fasting;
* Febrile;
* Xerostomic (such as in Sjögren's syndrome or after irradiation).

Superficial brown discoloration of the tongue and teeth (Figure 9.3), which is easily removed and of little consequence may be caused by:

* Cigarette smoking;
* Iron salts;
* Some foods and beverages (such as coffee and tea);
* Chlorhexidine;
* Amoxicillin.

Black and brown hairy tongue (Figures 9.4–9.6), appears to be caused by the elongation of the filiform papillae and accumulation of

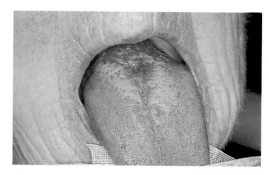

Figure 9.3
Brown hairy tongue

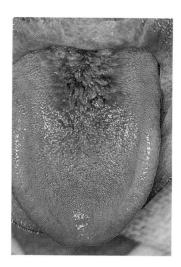

Figure 9.4
Black hairy tongue

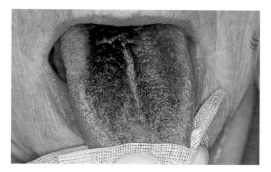

Figure 9.5
Black hairy tongue

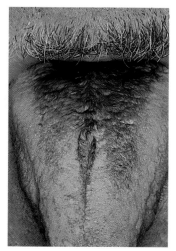

Figure 9.6
Black hairy tongue

epithelial squames and the proliferation of chromogenic microorganisms. It is seen particularly in:

- Drug abusers;
- Smokers;
- Alcohol drinkers;
- HIV infection.

Occasionally xerostomia or drugs are responsible, including:

- Antibiotics;

- Chlorhexidine;
- Corticosteroids;
- Griseofulvin;
- Lansoprazole;
- Monoamine oxidase inhibitors (MAOI);
- Methyldopa;
- Perborates;
- Peroxides;
- Phenothiazines;
- Tricyclics.

Clinical features

Brown or black hairy appearance of central dorsum of tongue, most severe posteriorly. The filiform papillae are excessively long and stained.

Diagnosis

Diagnosis is clear-cut.

Management

- Discontinue any drugs or mouthwashes responsible;
- Stop smoking;
- Increase the standard of oral hygiene;
- Scrape or brush the tongue with a toothbrush;
- Rarely, trim the hairs with scissors;
- Use sodium bicarbonate, peroxide or 40% urea in water mouthwashes;
- Chew pineapple and/or suck a peach stone;
- Caustic applications such as trichloracetic acid or podophyllum resin or retinoic acid (tretinoin; retin-A) may sometimes be needed in recalcitrant cases.

Burning mouth (tongue) syndrome

See Chapter 3

Candidal glossitis

Definition

Sore tongue caused by candidiasis

Incidence

Uncommon

Age mainly affected

Any

Sex mainly affected

M=F

Aetiology

Opportunistic infection with candida species, particularly *C. albicans*. Predisposing factors include the following:

- Broad-spectrum antimicrobials, particularly tetracycline;
- Topical corticosteroids (more often thrush);
- Xerostomia;
- Immune defects (more often thrush).

Clinical features

Diffuse erythema and soreness of tongue mainly (Figure 9.7). There may also be patches of thrush.

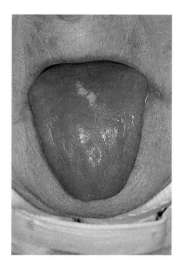

Figure 9.7
Candidal glossitis

Diagnosis

Diagnosis is mainly clinical but it may be helpful to smear for candidal hyphae or to take an oral rinse to assess degree of candidal infection.

Management

- Treat the predisposing cause;
- The patient should stop smoking;
- Give antifungals (Table 10.8).

Coated tongue (white hairy tongue)

A coated tongue (Figure 9.8) is a common problem, mainly in adults, due to collection of epithelial, food and microbial debris. The tongue is the main reservoir of microorganisms such as *Candida albicans* and some streptococci. Coating of the tongue is quite common in persons who are:

- Edentulous;
- On a soft, nonabrasive diet;
- Poor at oral hygiene;
- Fasting;
- Febrile;
- Xerostomic;
- Taking various medications.

It may be necessary to exclude other conditions such as thrush (rarely on dorsum of tongue), chronic candidiasis, hairy leukoplakia (lateral borders of tongue) or other leukoplakias, or a black hairy tongue.
   Treatment is:

- Treat the underlying condition;
- Improve oral hygiene;

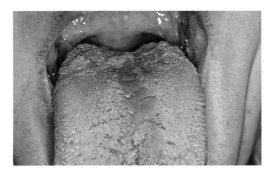

Figure 9.8
Coated tongue

- Brush the tongue;
- Use peroxide or ascorbic acid mouthwash.

Deficiency glossitis

Definition

Deficiency glossitis is a red, often sore, tongue due to haematinic deficiencies.

Incidence

Uncommon

Age mainly affected

Middle-aged and elderly

Sex mainly affected

M=F

Aetiology

Deficiencies of haematinics such as iron, folic acid, vitamin B12 (rarely other B vitamins). These deficiencies are uncommon except in malabsorption states, pernicious anaemia or the occasional vegan or other dietary faddist.

Clinical features

The sore tongue may:

- Appear normal;
- Show linear or patchy red lesions (especially in vitamin B12 deficiency; Figure 9.9);
- Be depapillated with erythema, termed glossitis (in deficiencies of iron, folic acid or B vitamins). Lingual depapillation begins at the tip and margins of the dorsum but later involves the whole dorsum (Figure 9.10);
- Be associated with oral ulceration, angular stomatitis or pallor.

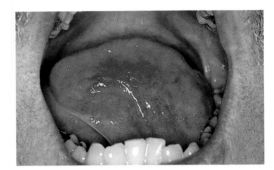

Figure 9.9
*Deficiency glossitis
showing erythematous
lesions*

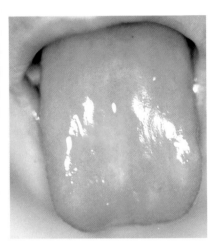

Figure 9.10
*Deficiency glossitis showing
complete depapillation*

Diagnosis

Haematological assays; haemoglobin, blood film, serum ferritin and vitamin B12 levels, and red cell folate levels.

Management

- Establish and rectify the underlying cause of the deficiency;
- Treat by replacement therapy.

Eosinophilic ulcer

Definition

Solitary ulcer that may resemble a carcinoma but contains prominent eosinophils, and is self-healing.

Incidence

Rare

Age mainly affected

Adults

Sex mainly affected

M=F

Aetiology

May be traumatic or reactive in origin.

Clinical features

- It is seen mainly on the dorsum or lateral margin of the tongue;
- Round or oval ulcer up to 3 cm in diameter;
- Persists for up to 8 weeks;
- Resembles a carcinoma clinically;
- Is self-healing.

Diagnosis

- Biopsy is often carried out because of the duration and resemblance to carcinoma;
- Haematology shows normal eosinophil count.

Management

This is self-healing but not infrequently is excised.

Erythema migrans (geographic tongue; benign migratory glossitis)

Definition

Red patches that change size and shape and resemble a map ('geographic'; Figure 9.11). Unrelated to the skin condition of the same name.

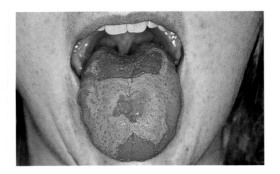

Figure 9.11
*Erythema migrans:
multiple depapillated
areas giving the
appearance of a map
(geographic tongue)*

Incidence

Common (affecting up to 2%)

Age mainly affected

Any

Sex mainly affected

F>M

Aetiology

It has a genetic background and a familial pattern is common.

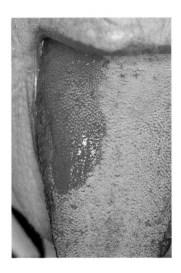

Figure 9.12
Erythema migrans

Clinical features

- It is seen mainly on the dorsum of the tongue (Figure 9.12);
- The filiform papillae desquamate in irregular demarcated areas, resulting in red patches of desquamation often with a yellow border (Figures 9.13–9.18);

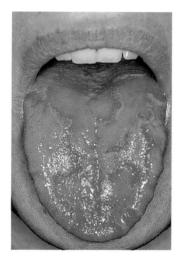

Figure 9.13
Erythema migrans

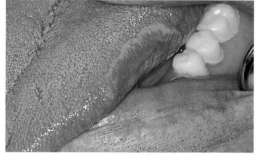

Figure 9.14
Erythema migrans: lesions may have yellowish border

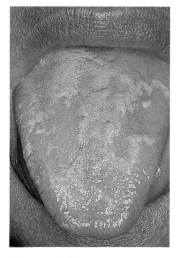

Figure 9.15
Erythema migrans

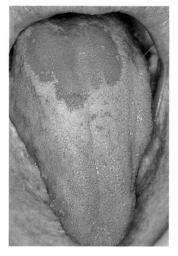

Figure 9.16
Erythema migrans

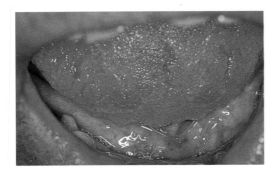

Figure 9.17
*Erythema migrans:
indistinct lesions*

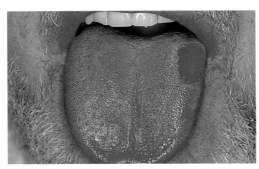

Figure 9.18
*Erythema migrans:
solitary lesion*

- The red areas change in shape, increase in size, and spread or move to other areas within hours;
- The condition may cause some soreness especially with acidic foods (e.g. tomatoes);
- Often found in patients who have a fissured tongue (Figures 9.19 and 9.20);
- Occasionally, similar lesions may appear elsewhere on the oral mucosa (Figure 9.21);
- Rarely there is an association with:
    - Pustular psoriasis;
    - Reiter's syndrome;
    - Atopic dermatitis;
    - Pityriasis rubra pilaris;
    - HIV infection.

Diagnosis

- The diagnosis is clinical;
- No investigations are usually needed unless there is the possibility of deficiency glossitis, Reiter's syndrome (transiently), psoriasis or other disorders.

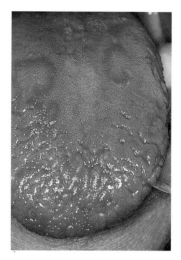

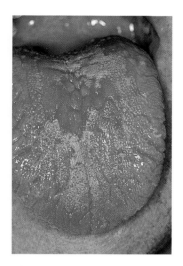

Figure 9.19
Erythema migrans

Figure 9.20
Erythema migrans in fissured tongue

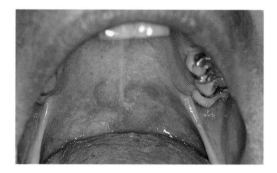

Figure 9.21
Erythema migrans

There also may be confusion with lichen planus and lupus erythematosus.

Management

The condition is not serious and there is no effective treatment. Zinc 200 mg three times daily for 3 months is advocated by some and may occasionally help. Reassurance is often all that can be offered.

Fissured tongue (scrotal or plicated tongue)

Definition

A tongue with fissures on the dorsum

Incidence

About 5% of the population

Age mainly affected

After puberty; the condition is more noticeable with increasing age.

Sex mainly affected

M=F

Aetiology

Fissured tongue is:

- A common developmental anomaly;
- Of little significance;
- Often associated with erythema migrans;
- One feature of Melkersson–Rosenthal syndrome (see page 189);
- Found more frequently than normal in Down's syndrome;
- Found more frequently than normal in psoriasis.

Clinical features

There are multiple fissures on the dorsum of the tongue (Figures 9.19 and 9.22), and it may be complicated by geographic tongue. Otherwise it is asymptomatic.

Diagnosis

The diagnosis is usually clear-cut, though the lobulated tongue of Sjögren's syndrome and chronic mucocutaneous candidiasis (Figure 9.23) must be differentiated.

Management

Reassure the patient.

Foliate papillitis

The size and shape of the foliate papillae on the postero-lateral margins of the tongue are variable. These papillae occasionally swell if irritated mechanically or if there is an upper respiratory infection.

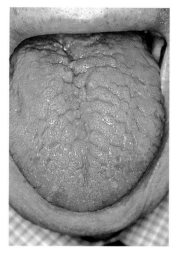

Figure 9.22
Fissured tongue

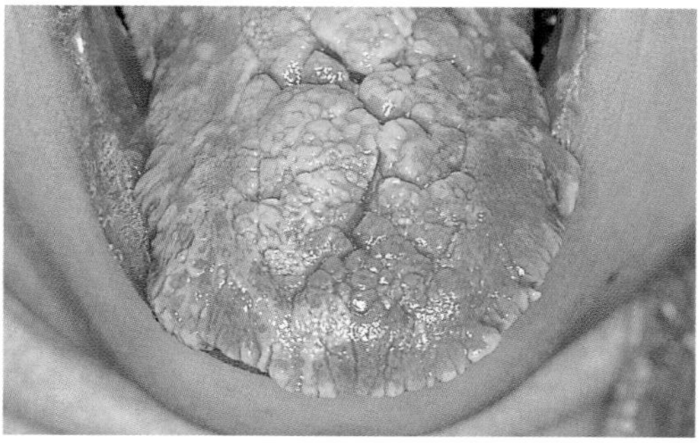

Figure 9.23
*Chronic mucocutaneous candidiasis:
the tongue often becomes fissured*

Located at a site of high predilection for lingual cancer, they may give rise to anxiety about cancer.

Geographic tongue

See erythema migrans

Glossodynia

See Chapter 3

Granular cell tumour

Definition

A solitary tumour in which granular cells are prominent

Incidence

Uncommon

Age mainly affected

Adult

Sex mainly affected

F>M

Aetiology

Idiopathic. Arises from Schwann cells, which stain for S100 and vimentin.

Clinical features

- Solitary, slow-growing asymptomatic swelling;
- Most common in tongue;
- Appears to have a small malignant predisposition (<1%).

Diagnosis

- Clinical;
- Biopsy; this shows granular cells and pseudocarcinomatous hyperplasia.

Management

- Excise;
- Reassure the patient.

Hairy leukoplakia

See Chapter 4

Definition

Bilateral white lesions on the tongue, usually in an immunocompromised individual, mainly in AIDS.

Incidence

Uncommon

Age mainly affected

Adult

Sex mainly affected

M>F

Aetiology

Epstein–Barr virus, usually in an immunocompromised patient

Clinical features

- White lesions on both sides of the tongue, vertically corrugated (Figures 9.24 and 9.25);
- Appears to have no premalignant predisposition;
- Appears to be benign, and self-limiting.

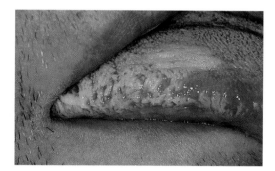

Figure 9.24
Hairy leukoplakia in AIDS

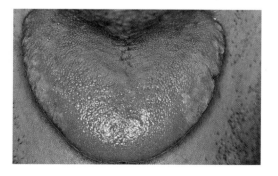

Figure 9.25
Hairy leukoplakia

Diagnosis

- Clinical;
- HIV serotest;
- Sometimes biopsy, probing for EBV.

Management

- Reassure the patient;
- Antiretroviral and antiherpes agents may clear the lesion.

Hairy tongue

See page 360

Lingual thyroid

This is a small sessile lump, seen mainly in females, in the midline of the tongue posterior to the foramen caecum. It can cause dysphagia, dysphonia and occasionally dyspnoea. The neck should be examined and a scan performed to ensure there is a normal thyroid before such lump is excised (Figure 9.26). However, midline lumps in the posterior tongue rarely prove to be due to a lingual thyroid.

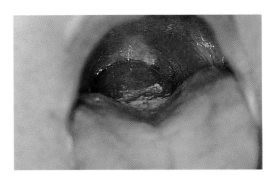

Figure 9.26
Lingual thyroid

Median rhomboid glossitis

Definition

This is a depapillated rhomboidal area in the centre line of the dorsum of tongue anterior to the circumvallate papillae.

Incidence

Uncommon

Age mainly affected

Adults

Sex mainly affected

M>F

Aetiology

Previously considered developmental, now candidal. Usually the patient is a smoker. A similar lesion may be seen in HIV disease, or precipitated by corticosteroids.

Clinical features

- Depapillated rhomboidal area in the centre line of the dorsum of tongue anterior to circumvallate papillae (Figures 9.27–9.30);
- Flat or nodular, red, or red and white;
- Usually asymptomatic.

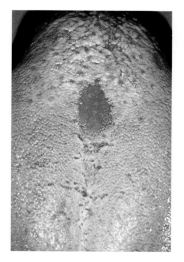

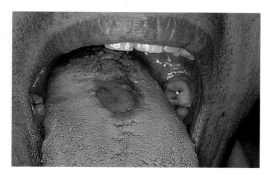

Figure 9.28
Median rhomboid glossitis

Figure 9.27
Median rhomboid glossitis

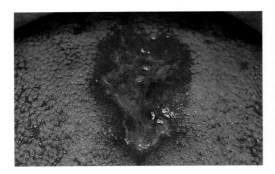

Figure 9.29
Median rhomboid glossitis

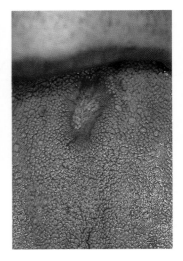

Figure 9.30
Median rhomboid glossitis

Diagnosis

Biopsy is not usually needed as the location is typical and tumours are rare at this site. Histology however, may show pseudocarcinomatous features.

Management

- The patient should stop smoking;
- Antifungals may be indicated, often for several weeks or months (Table 10.8);
- Cryosurgery may be required if the lesion does not resolve.

Oral–facial–digital syndrome

Multiple fibrous bands may be associated with cleft or lobulated tongue, oral–facial–digital syndrome (OFD).

- OFD type I, seen only in girls, includes also clinodactyly, cleft palate and sometimes renal defects;
- OFD type II is less severe but there is often also conductive deafness.

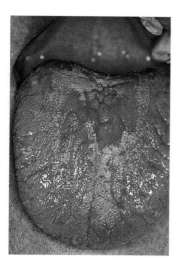

Figure 9.31
Erythema migrans in a fissured tongue; a common combination causing sore tongue

Soreness

Soreness of the tongue is not uncommon and a lesion cannot always be seen. Important causes include erythema migrans (Figure 9.31), burning mouth syndrome (Chapter 3), ulcers of any cause, deficiency glossitis, lichen planus and candidiasis.

Sublingual keratosis

Definition

Sublingual keratosis is a white plaque in the sublingual region.

Incidence

Uncommon

Age mainly affected

Middle-aged and elderly

Sex mainly affected

M=F

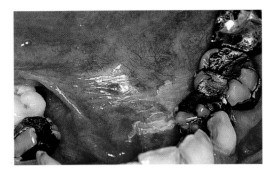

Figure 9.32
Sublingual (floor of mouth) keratosis

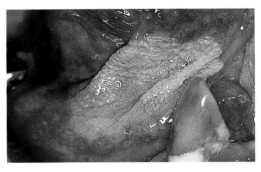

Figure 9.33
Sublingual (floor of mouth) keratosis

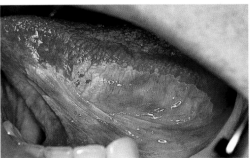

Figure 9.34
Sublingual (floor of mouth) keratosis

Aetiology

Idiopathic. Formerly thought to be congenital

Clinical features

The features include (Figures 4.120, 4.121 and 9.32–9.34):

- White plaque;
- Location in the sublingual region. The plaque typically is bilateral and extends from the anterior floor of the mouth onto the

undersurface of the tongue. Those on the lingual ventrum alone may be unilateral;

- Wrinkled surface;
- An irregular but well-defined outline and sometimes a butterfly shape;
- No induration.

This lesion was formerly categorized as a benign epithelial naevus but malignant change was associated in 24% of less than 30 cases reported about 20 years ago. Such a high risk of malignant change however, has not been widely confirmed and a figure of 15% may be more realistic.

Diagnosis

Diagnosis is clinical but for the above reasons, biopsy may be indicated.

Management

Opinions vary as to whether the lesion should be left undisturbed or removed surgically by scalpel, electrosurgery, laser or cryoprobe.

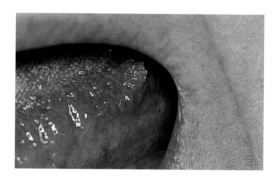

Figure 9.35
Papilloma

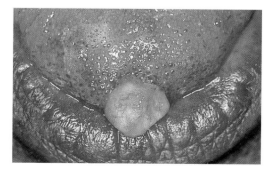

Figure 9.36
Fibrous lump

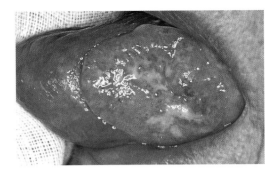

Figure 9.37
Carcinoma in the most common intraoral site, the lateral margin of the tongue posteriorly

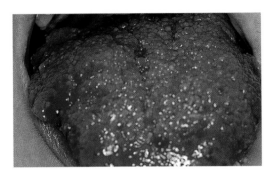

Figure 9.38
Lymphangioma

Swelling

Discrete lumps of the tongue may be of various causes:

- Congenital: lingual thyroid, haemangioma, lymphangioma;
- Neoplastic: papilloma (Figure 9.35), fibrous lump (Figures 4.152 and 9.36), carcinoma (Figure 9.37), granular cell tumour (granular cell myoblastoma), Kaposi's sarcoma;
- Traumatic: oedema, haematoma, foreign body;
- Cysts;
- Inflammatory: infection, abscess.

Generalized swelling (macroglossia) may be congenital:
- Down's syndrome;
- Lymphangioma (Figure 9.38);
- Haemangioma;
- Beckwith–Wiedemann syndrome;
- Neurofibromatosis;
- Multiple endocrine adenomatosis;
- Cretinism;
- Hurler's syndrome (mucopolysaccharidosis);
- Hereditary angioedema.

Or acquired:
- Inflammatory oedema;
- Angioedema;
- Gigantism;
- Acromegaly;
- Amyloidosis;
- Other rare causes.

Microglossia:
- Aglossia–adactylia syndrome;
- Moebius' syndrome.

Syphilitic leukoplakia

Definition

White mucosal lesion in tertiary syphilis

Incidence

Rare

Age mainly affected

Middle-aged and elderly

Sex mainly affected

M>F

Aetiology

Leukoplakia of the dorsum of the tongue is a characteristic complication of tertiary syphilis but is now rare.

Clinical features

Syphilitic leukoplakia had no distinctive features, but typically affected the dorsum of the tongue and spared the margins (Figure 9.39). The lesion had an irregular outline and surface. It was usually

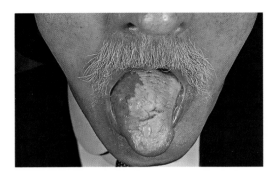

Figure 9.39
Syphilitic leukoplakia

regarded as having a high risk of malignant change and cracks, small erosions or nodules which may be foci or carcinoma.

Diagnosis

Serology for syphilis, and biopsy

Management

Antibiotics

Further reading

Brooks JK, Balciunas BA. Geographical stomatitis: review of the literature and report of five cases. *J Am Dent Assoc* (1987) **115**: 421–4.

Browning S, Hislop S, Scully C, Shirlaw P. The association between burning mouth syndrome and psychosocial disorders. *Oral Surg Oral Med Oral Pathol* (1987) **64**: 171–4.

Collo D. Differentialdiagnose der Makroglossie. *Dtsch Arztebl* (1975) **39**: 2693–8.

Kullaa-Mikkonen A. Familial study of fissured tongue. *Scand J Dent Res* (1988) **96**: 366–75.

Langtry JA, Carr MM, Steele MC, Ive FA. Topical tretinoin: a new treatment for black hairy tongue (lingua villosa nigra). *Clin Exp Dermatol* (1992) **17**: 163–4.

Notestine GE. The importance of the identification of ankyloglossia (short lingual frenulum) as a cause of breastfeeding problems. *J Hum Lact* (1990) **6**: 113–15.

Sarti GM et al. Black hairy tongue. *Am Fam Physician* (1990) **41**: 1751.

Toume LPM, Fricton JR. Burning mouth syndrome. *Oral Surg Oral Med Oral Pathol* (1992) **74**: 158–67.

van der Waal N, van der Kwast WA, van der Waal I. Median rhomboid glossitis: a follow-up study of 16 patients. *J Oral Med* (1986) **41**: 117–20.

Diagnosis and treatment

Certain management procedures are commonplace and therefore discussed here.

Diagnosis

The purpose of making a diagnosis is to be able to offer the:

- Most effective treatment;
- Safest treatment;
- Most accurate prognostication.

History

Diagnosis most importantly involves a careful history; the patient will
often deliver the diagnosis from the history. A relevant medical history
is also extremely important. Due cognisance must always be taken of
the cultural and social background of the patient when taking the history.

Examination

Dental staff should:

- Enquire about extraoral lesions;
- Observe the patient's affect, behaviour, movements and gait;
- Inspect and examine the hands, fingers, nails, wrists (and pulse),
  face and neck and cervical lymph nodes.

A careful inspection and examination of the oral and perioral structures is mandatory, always commencing in the area most remote from

that of which the patient complains, in order not to miss other lesions.

A full physical examination must be carried out if there is any possibility of systemic disease but is not appropriate in most dental practice; again, the cultural background may dictate what is possible. Specialist referral may be indicated for full extraoral examination.

Investigations

Investigations may help the diagnosis and possibly prognosis.
Inadequate investigation could:

- Lead to a misdiagnosis;
- Lead to a missed diagnosis;
- Be regarded as bad practice;
- Result in a legal action.

Superfluous investigations are:

- Liable to engender undue anxiety on the part of the patient, partner or relatives;
- Time consuming;
- Expensive;
- Sometimes dangerous.

The potential benefits from investigations and of *not* carrying out the investigations have always to be weighed against possible adverse effects, and both should be explained to the patient. Informed consent is mandatory for all investigations involving operative procedures and care must be taken not to produce anxiety where it is not necessary.

Patients not uncommonly complain that they have been ill-informed about their diagnosis, investigations and the results of these. Whether or not this is true, it is the duty of dental staff to ensure they try to help patients understand their condition. One way to help, in addition to personal discussion, is by writing important points down for the patient, and using Patient Information Sheets; examples are included in this book.

Blood tests, radiographs or other investigations may be needed.

Biopsy

Biopsy is often indicated in order to establish the precise diagnosis, especially in the case of mucosal lesions, and a specimen for immunostaining is increasingly called for. Some patients equate biopsy with a diagnosis of cancer and so should be managed tactfully.

Complete the request form with the patient's full name, hospital number if applicable, date, site of biopsy, clinical résumé, and dates and numbers of all previous biopsies.

The container must be labelled clearly with patient's full name, number, date and specimen site.

Biopsy technique

Mucosal biopsies are *excisional* (removal of the complete lesion), taken usually with a scalpel, or *incisional* and taken with a scalpel or punch, usually under local analgesia, or taken with a special brush to remove cells.

The scalpel or punch biopsy should include lesional and normal tissue. In the case of ulcerated mucosal lesions, most histopathological information is gleaned from the perilesional tissue since by definition most epithelium is lost from the ulcer itself (Figures 10.1 and 10.2). The punch has the advantage that the incision is controlled, the patient is not disturbed by the sight of a scalpel, and suturing may not be required. However, only a fairly small biopsy is obtained and, in some instances, a larger piece of tissue is needed. A 6 mm or 4 mm punch should be used. In the case of a suspected potentially malignant or malignant lesion, vital staining may be indicated to highlight the area to biopsy.

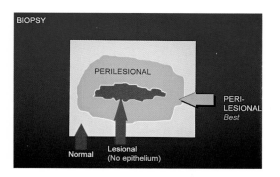

Figure 10.1
Biopsy of mucosal ulcer; perilesional tissue should be taken

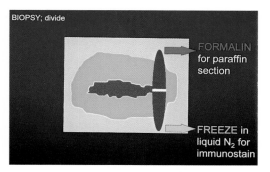

Figure 10.2
Biopsy specimens required when examining mucosal lesions

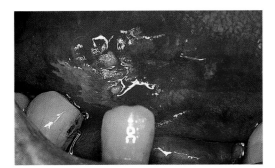

Figure 10.3
Vital staining; lesion before toluidine blue staining

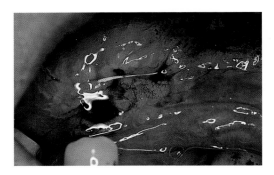

Figure 10.4
Vital staining; lesion after toluidine blue staining, highlighting areas best for biopsy

Vital staining

In the case of suspected potentially malignant or malignant lesions it can be difficult to decide exactly which area is best biopsied. Most significant information can be gained from red areas rather than white areas and it can be helpful to stain the mucosa prebiopsy with toluidine blue dye, which is taken up and stains pathological areas mainly (Figures 10.3 and 10.4). The usual procedure is for:

- The patient to rinse for 20 seconds with a solution of acetic acid to cleanse the area of mucus, etc.;
- The patient to rinse for 20 seconds with water;
- The patient to rinse for 60 seconds with a toluidine blue (tolonium blue) solution;
- The patient to rinse for 20 seconds with a poststaining solution of acetic acid;
- The patient to rinse for 20 seconds with water.

Suspect areas stain blue.

To carry out biopsy, a local analgesic should be given and then:

- Include some normal tissue as well as the lesion (biopsies of ulcers alone are inadequate);

- Do not squeeze with forceps. Sutures may be used to hold the tissue and also to mark specific areas of biopsy;
- Place tissue on to a small piece of paper before immersing in fixative, to prevent curling;
- Suture if necessary.

Histology

Put small specimens immediately into buffered formalin or other fixative in at least its own volume of fixative. Put large specimens into fixative in plastic bags. Leave formalin-fixed specimens at room temperature.

If bacteriological examination is required, for example in suspected tuberculosis, send a separate specimen without fixative.

Immunology

Specimens are not usually fixed, but immediately snap-frozen (on solid CO_2 or liquid nitrogen). A further biopsy specimen (or half of a larger biopsy) should be immediately snap-frozen.

Lymph node

Lymph nodes should not be subjected to open biopsy if malignant disease is suspected; fine needle aspiration biopsy (FNAB) is better or the biopsy deferred until time of operation.

Lymph nodes have a blood supply that must be ligated before incision. Lymph nodes are often closely related to large veins and sometimes large arteries. Some lymph nodes are closely related to important nerves. Some pathologists like to make an imprint from the fresh cut surface of lymph nodes. They may wish to do this personally. Make an adequate skin incision. Do not squeeze the node or fragment it, but remove it whole. Put it straight into fixative, unless some is needed for culture or guinea pig inoculation.

Labial salivary gland (page 7, Figure 1.6)

- Make a linear mucosal incision (midline in lower labial mucosa, towards the sulcus);
- Excise at least four lobules of salivary gland;
- Suture if necessary.

Frozen sections for rapid diagnosis

Communicate with the pathologist at the latest by the day before the operation. Telephone the laboratory when the specimen is on its way.

Warn the pathologist about any tissue containing calcified material *before* he breaks his microtome.

Oral smears for cytology

- Take smears with a wooden or metal spatula, or dental plastic instrument;
- Spread evenly on the centres of two previously labelled glass slides;
- Fix immediately in industrial methylated spirit. Do not allow to dry in air, as cellular detail is rapidly lost and artefacts develop;
- After 20 minutes of fixation, the smears can then be left to dry in the air or left in fixative.

Prepared in this way, smears will keep for up to 3 weeks.

These procedures can often be carried out in practice but, for a number of reasons, the dental surgeon may elect to refer to a specialist. The same applies to other investigations, particularly where there are sensitive issues such as possible HIV infection, where medical experience or a medical or specialist opinion would be helpful if not essential.

Management

Oral hygiene

Dental staff should also ensure the patient has appropriate oral health education, and maintains particularly good oral hygiene, since the limited evidence available suggests that good oral hygiene helps the resolution of some mucosal lesions (Table 10.1). Antiplaque agents such as chlorhexidine are thus commonly used, particularly if the patient is immunocompromised.

Diet

Many mucosal lesions are aggravated by irritants such as tobacco and alcohol, and these also decrease salivary flow and should thus be avoided. In contrast, a healthy balanced diet is indicated to help resolution of mucosal lesions in particular. Puréed nonirritant foods and avoiding toast and potato crisps, spices, and acids such as in tomatoes and citrus fruits, may be indicated for a short period whilst a patient has a sore mouth. Dietary control is essential in xerostomia, to avoid caries.

Treatment of oral lesions

Medical conditions are not always amenable to cure. Control of symptoms, however, is usually achievable. The beneficial effect of a supportive and understanding clinician is often underestimated.

Table 10.1   Some mouthwashes with antimicrobial activity

Agent	Dose	Comments*
Chlorhexidine gluconate	0.1–0.2% aqueous mouthwash, rinse for 1 min twice daily. Also gel or spray	Has significant antiplaque activity. May stain teeth if patient drinks tea or coffee
Povidone iodide	1% mouthwash used twice to four times daily for up to 14 days	Contraindicated in iodine sensitivity, pregnancy, thyroid disorders or those taking lithium
Cetylpyridinium chloride	0.05% mouthwash used twice daily	
Hexetidine	0.1% mouthwash used twice daily	

*All occasionally may cause mucosal irritation.

- The first principle must be to do no harm;
- It is important to discuss the condition and possible therapy with the patient concerned, and warn of likely consequences (good and bad) of treatment or no treatment, and of possible adverse reactions;
- All surgery is invasive;
- Only the operator adequately skilled in a procedure should perform it;
- Most drugs can have adverse effects;
- Prescribe only drugs with which you are totally familiar;
- Ensure there is no history of allergy or untoward effect;
- Always check drug doses, contraindications, interactions and adverse reactions;
- Reduce drug doses in children, the elderly, liver disease and kidney disease;
- Where possible, drugs should be avoided in pregnancy.

Analgesia

Specific treatments for many orofacial lesions are few and far between, and often all that can be offered is an agent to reduce the inflammatory response, or relieve discomfort or pain, and compassion. Erosive or ulcerative lesions can be protected with *Orabase* or *Zilactin*.

Topical agents with analgesic actions may be helpful (Table 10.2). A variety of 'over the counter' (OTC) preparations is also available though few have been proved effective in controlled trials.

Table 10.2   Agents which may reduce pain from mucosal lesions

Agent	Use	Comments
Benzydamine hydrochloride	Rinse or spray every 1.5–3 hours	Effective in reducing discomfort in radiation mucositis
Carboxymethylcellulose	Paste or powder used after meals to protect area	Available containing triamcinolone
Lignocaine (Lidocaine)	Topical 4% solution may ease pain	

Pain is the most important symptom suggestive of oral disease but absence of pain does not exclude disease. There is considerable individual variation in response to pain, and the threshold is lowered by tiredness, and psychogenic and other factors. It is important where possible to:

- Identify and treat the cause of pain;
- Relieve factors that lower the pain threshold (fatigue, anxiety and depression).

Try simple analgesics, before embarking on more potent preparations and avoid polypharmacy (Table 10.3). Simple analgesics such as paracetamol may be required and in children can be usefully given in sugar-free syrups. Aspirin is often used but it is a nonsteroidal anti-inflammatory drug (NSAID) and thus can:

- Cause peptic ulceration and further deterioration of renal function, if this is already impaired;
- Worsen asthma;
- Cause fluid retention;
- Cause nausea, diarrhoea or tinnitus;
- Increase methotrexate toxicity;
- Interfere with antihypertensives and diuretics.

Aspirin has been longer in use than most NSAIDs, and the efficacy and adverse effects are well recognized. The same comments cannot be said to apply to all of the newer agents. However, aspirin should be avoided in:

- Children under the age of 12 years (possible association with Reye's syndrome, a serious liver disease);
- Mothers who are breast feeding (passes in milk to child);
- Gastric disease (possible ulceration);
- Bleeding tendency (interferes with platelet function).

Table 10.3   Analgesics

Agent	Dosage	Contraindications
Nonsteroidal anti-inflammatory drugs (NSAIDs)		
Mefenamic acid	250–500 mg up to 3 times a day	Asthma, gastrointestinal, renal and liver disease, pregnancy
Diflunisal	250–500 mg twice a day	Pregnancy, peptic ulcer, allergies, renal and liver disease
NonNSAIDs		
Paracetamol	500–1000 mg up to 6 times a day (max 4 mg daily)	Liver or renal disease or those on zidovudine
Nefopam	30–60 mg up to 3 times a day	Convulsive disorders, pregnancy, elderly, renal, liver disease
Opioids		
Codeine	10–60 mg up to 6 times a day (or 30 mg intramuscularly)	Late pregnancy and liver disease
Dihydrocodeine	30 mg up to 4 times a day (or 50 mg intramuscularly)	Children, hypothyroidism asthma, renal disease
Pentazocine	25–50 mg up to 4 times a day (or 30 mg intramuscularly or intravenously)	Pregnancy, children, hypertension, respiratory depression, head injuries or raised intracranial pressure

Paracetamol (acetaminophen) is often more useful since it is not an NSAID and produces no platelet dysfunction. Chronic pain requires regular analgesia (not just as 'required') and it is important not to overdose with paracetamol which is hepatotoxic in high doses.

Reassurance is often remarkably effective at calming the anxious patient but there are times when a mild anxiolytic can be helpful (Table 10.4).

Immunosuppressive and immunomodulatory agents

Topical corticosteroids are useful in the management of many oral ulcerative conditions where there is no systemic involvement, such as recurrent aphthous stomatitis and lichen planus (Table 10.5). With many topical steroids there is little systemic absorption and thus no significant adrenocortical suppression. Creams, gels and inhalers are better than ointments since these adhere poorly to the mucosa.

Table 10.4   Anxiolytics

Drug	Dose	Comments
Diazepam		Avoid in glaucoma
	2–30 mg daily in divided doses	Use with caution in the elderly
Temazepam		Avoid in glaucoma
	5–10 mg at night	Use with caution in the elderly

Table 10.5   Examples of topical corticosteroids

Steroid	Dosage every 6 hours	Comments
Hydrocortisone hemisuccinate pellets	2.5 mg dissolve in mouth close to ulcers	Use at an early stage of recurrent aphthous stomatitis
Triamcinolone acetonide in carmellose gelatin paste	Apply to lesions	Adheres best to dry mucosa; affords mechanical protection; of little benefit on tongue or palate
More potent		
Betamethasone phosphate tablets	0.5 mg; use as mouthwash	May produce adrenal suppression
Beclomethasone spray	1 puff 100 µg	May produce adrenal suppression
Budesonide spray	1 puff 100 µg	May produce adrenal suppression
Fluocinolone	Apply to lesion	May produce adrenal suppression
Fluocinonide cream gel or ointment	Apply to lesion	May produce adrenal suppression
Highly potent		
Clobetasol cream	Apply to lesion	May produce adrenal suppression
Prednisolone mouthwash	5 mg	May produce adrenal suppression

Patients should not eat or drink for 30 minutes after using the steroid, in order to prolong contact with the lesion. The steroid can usefully be applied in a plastic splint worn overnight for treatment of desquamative gingivitis. In patients using potent steroids for more than a month it is prudent to add an antifungal, since candidiasis may arise.

Intralesional corticosteroids are occasionally useful in the management of intractable local lesions, such as erosive lichen planus

Table 10.6   Intralesional corticosteroids

Prednisolone sodium phosphate: up to 22 mg
Methylprednisolone acetate: 4–80 mg
Triamcinolone acetonide: 2–3 mg
Triamcinolone hexacetonide: up to 5 mg

(see Table 10.6). Intra-articular corticosteroids are occasionally indicated where there is intractable pain from a noninfective arthropathy.

Systemic corticosteroids are often indicated for the management of:

- Pemphigus;
- Giant cell arteritis;
- Bell's palsy;
- Multisystem diseases such as lichen planus with oral, genital and cutaneous involvement;
- Severe or resistant oral ulceration in vesiculobullous conditions.

Systemic corticosteroids must always be used with caution.

- Adrenocortical suppression makes the patient liable to collapse if they are stressed, traumatized or have an infection;
- Patients should always be given a steroid card, warned of possible adverse reactions, and warned of the need for an increase in the dose if ill, traumatized, or having an operation;
- Hypertension and precipitation of diabetes are other important effects; the blood pressure and glucose must always be monitored;
- Psychoses and osteoporosis are other serious complications;
- Patients on steroids are, by definition, immunosuppressed and liable to infections, especially with viruses and fungi;
- Alternate day administration reduces the adverse effects of steroids;
- A 'steroid sparing' effect can be achieved with drugs such as azathioprine (Table 10.7), cyclosporin, tacrolimus, levamisole, colchicine, thalidomide, dapsone or pentoxifylline. However, these have other, sometimes more serious, adverse effects and should be reserved for specialist use.

Retinoids

Tretinoin as a 0.1% cream or 0.01% gel, or etretinate orally 50–75 mg daily, may be of value in controlling lichen planus. Systemic retinoids are teratogenic.

Table 10.7 Systemic immunosuppressants and immunomodulatory agents

Drug	Dose	Comments*	Main indications
Prednisolone	Initially 40–80 mg orally each day in divided doses, reducing as soon as possible to 10 mg daily (give as enteric coated prednisolone with meals)	Limit dosage in hypertension and diabetes mellitus. See text for adverse effects	Pemphigus Other severe or widespread vesiculobullous disorders Behcet's syndrome Bell's palsy Giant cell arteritis
Azathioprine	2–2.5 mg/kg daily	May cause bone marrow suppression, liver dysfunction, arrhythmias, hypotension, nephritis Contraindicated in pregnancy	Pemphigus, pemphigoid
Colchicine	500 μg, 3 times daily	Causes diarrhoea and bone marrow suppression Contraindicated in pregnancy, elderly, cardiac, renal or hepatic disease	Behcet's syndrome EB acquisita
Dapsone	1 mg/kg/day	Causes haemolysis and methaemoglobinaemia Contraindicated in G6PD deficiency, (monitor reticulocyte count closely) pregnancy, cardiorespiratory disease	Pemphigoid, linear IgA disease Behcet's syndrome
Cyclosporin (Ciclosporin)	1–2 mg/kg/day	Nephrotoxic. May cause hypertension, blood dyscrasias Contraindicated in kidney disease, pregnancy, porphyria	Lichen planus, pemphigus, pemphigoid, Behcet's syndrome
Cyclophosphamide	1–2 mg/kg/day	Can cause bone marrow suppression, cystitis, neoplasms	Pemphigus, pemphigoid Wegener's granulomatosis, Behcet's syndrome
Thalidomide	100–200 mg daily	Teratogenic Neurotoxic	Behcet's syndrome, severe aphthae, ulcers in HIV disease
Pentoxifylline (Oxpentifylline)	400 mg twice daily	Contraindicated in cerebrovascular haemorrhage, myocardial infarction	

*Most can increase liability to infection, and in the long term possibly also neoplasia.

Hydroxychloroquine

Hydroxychloroquine 200–400 mg daily may, after some months control lichen planus or lupus erythematosus. Ophthalmic monitoring is necessary.

Antimicrobials

Drainage must be established if there is pus; antimicrobials will not remove pus. A sample of pus (as much as possible) should be sent for culture and sensitivities but, if antimicrobials are indicated, they should be started immediately and in adequate doses.

Anaerobes are responsible for many odontogenic infections, and these often respond to penicillins or metronidazole. Very high blood antimicrobial levels can now be achieved with oral amoxycillin, with good patient compliance. If the patient is allergic, or has had penicillin with the previous month (resistant bacteria) another antimicrobial should be used.

If a lesion fails to respond to an antimicrobial reconsider possible:

- Inadequacy of drainage;
- Inappropriateness of the antimicrobial;
- Inadequate antimicrobial dose;
- Antimicrobial insensitivity of causal microorganism. For example, staphylococci are now frequently resistant to penicillin and some show multiple resistances, e.g. MRSA (methicillin-resistant *Staphylococcus aureus*);
- Patient noncompliance;
- Local factors (e.g. foreign body);
- Unusual type of infection;
- Impaired host defences (unusual and opportunistic infections are increasingly identified, particularly in the immunocompromised patient);
- Noninfective cause for the condition.

In serious, unusual or unresponsive cases of infection, consult the clinical microbiologist.

Antifungals (Table 10.8)

Antifungals are used to treat oral or oropharyngeal fungal infections but underlying predisposing factors should be corrected first.

Antifungal resistance to the azoles (ketoconazole, fluconazole, miconazole, itraconazole) is now becoming a significant problem for

Table 10.8 Antifungals

Agent	Dosage and duration (continue for at least 48 h after lesions have cleared)*	Possible drug interactions and contraindications†
Chlorhexidine	0.12–0.2% mouthrinse twice daily	Tooth staining especially if the patient drinks tea or coffee
Amphotericin	10 mg lozenge 100 mg/ml suspension 10–400 mg 6 hourly for at least 14–21 days	Topical use; no problems
Amphotericin (intravenous)	0.5 mg/kg for at least 10–14 days	Nephrotoxicity, arrhythmias, neuropathies, anaphylactoid reactions. Liposomal amphotericin may be safer Avoid in pregnancy. Expensive
Nystatin (topical)	500 000 unit lozenge 100 000 unit pastille 100 000 units per ml of suspension 100 000 units 6 hourly for at least 14–21 days	Topical use; often no problems but may cause unpleasant taste, nausea or gastrointestinal disturbance. Suspension contains sucrose
Clotrimazole (topical)	10 mg 6 hourly for at least 14 days	Not available in the UK. Difficult to dissolve if mouth dry. Contains sucrose.
Miconazole	250 mg tablet	Even topical agent may be absorbed systemically. May interact with many drugs including antidiabetics, anticoagulants, phenytoin, midazolam, cyclosporin, cisapride and astemizole.
(topical)	25 mg/ml gel 250 mg 6 hourly for at least 14–21 days	Avoid in pregnancy, porphyria

Drug	Dose	Notes
Ketoconazole (oral)	50 mg/g denture lacquer; apply weekly for at least 2 weeks 200–400 mg daily for at least 14 days	May impair oral contraceptive Not absorbed in achlorhydria. Hepatotoxic. Expensive. May interact with many drugs including anticoagulants, phenytoin, midazolam, cyclosporin, sertindole, terfenadine, cisapride and astemizole. Avoid in pregnancy, porphyria. May impair oral contraceptive
Fluconazole (oral)	50–200 mg daily for at least 14 days	May interact with drugs including antidiabetics, anticoagulants, phenytoin, midazolam, cyclosporin, zidovudine, terfenadine, cisapride and astemizole. Avoid in pregnancy, porphyria. May sometimes be hepatotoxic and myelosuppressive. Expensive. May impair oral contraceptive
Itraconazole (oral)	100–200 mg daily for at least 14 days 10 mg/ml liquid 10 ml twice daily for at least 14 days	Not absorbed in achlorhydria. May interact with many drugs including digoxin, sertindole, anticoagulants, phenytoin, midazolam, cyclosporin, simvastatin, terfenadine, cisapride and astemizole. Avoid in pregnancy, porphyria. Expensive. May impair oral contraceptive

•The higher doses are used in HIV infection.
†Check pharmacopoiea for other contraindications, cautions and interactions.

immunocompromised persons, especially those with a severe immune defect, who may show candida species resistant to fluconazole and, sometimes, to other azoles.

Azoles may displace protein-bound drugs and thus enhance the activity of, for example, anticoagulants, producing a bleeding tendency. Azoles may also interact with a number of drugs, and an important interaction is to produce arrhythmias with terfenadine, astemizole and cisapride. They may also interfere with the oral contraceptive pill.

Antivirals

There are few antiviral agents of proven efficacy. Some antiherpes agents are available. Most will achieve maximum benefit if given early in the disease. Immunocompromised patients with viral infections may well benefit from active antiviral therapy, since these infections may otherwise spread locally and systematically (see Table 10.9).

Antiviral resistance is now becoming a significant problem to immunocompromised persons, especially those with a severe immune defect, who may show herpesviruses resistant to aciclovir and, sometimes, to other antivirals.

Table 10.9   Antiviral therapy of oral viral infections in the immunocompromised

Disorder	Drug/dosage
Herpes simplex stomatitis	Aciclovir 100–200 mg tablets 5 times daily, or oral suspension (200 mg/5 ml) 5 times daily, or intravenously 250 mg/m^2 every 8 hours
Recurrent herpes	Aciclovir as above or penciclovir 1% cream every 2 hours or 5% aciclovir cream every 2 hours
Herpes varicella zoster	Aciclovir 800 mg oral 5 times daily, or aciclovir intravenously 500 mg/m^2 (5 mg/kg) every 8 hours, or famciclovir 250 mg 3 times daily, or famciclovir 750 mg once daily

Aciclovir (systemic preparations): caution in renal disease and pregnancy. Occasional increase in liver enzymes and urea, rashes, CNS effects.
Famciclovir: caution in renal disease and pregnancy. Occasionally causes nausea and headache.

Antidepressants (see Table 10.10)

Drugs are used for the treatment of depression but, psychotherapy and possibly physical treatment are also required. Only limited amounts of

Table 10.10   Some antidepressants

Drug	Dose	Comments
Amitriptyline	25–75 mg daily divided dose	Contraindicated in recent myocardial infarction, arrhythmias, liver disease
Dothiepin (Dosulepin)	25 mg 3 times a day or 75 mg at night	Contraindicated in recent myocardial infarction, arrhythmias, liver disease
Doxepine	25 mg 3 times a day or 75 mg at night	Contraindicated in recent myocardial infarction, arrhythmias, liver disease
Clomipramine	10–100 mg daily in divided doses	Contraindicated in recent myocardial infarction, arrhythmias, liver disease
Fluoxetine	20 mg daily	Caution with epilepsy, pregnancy, cardiac, liver, kidney disease, allergy or mania

antidepressants should be prescribed, as there is a danger that the patient may use them in a suicide attempt. There may be up to 3–4 weeks before the antidepressant action takes place. Monitoring of plasma concentrations of the drug may be helpful in ensuring optimal dosage. The natural history of depression is of remission after 3–12 months. Do not withdraw antidepressants prematurely. Doses should be reduced for the elderly patient. If there is any possibility of a suicide attempt the patient must be seen by a psychiatrist as a matter of urgency.

Points to bear in mind are that:

- Antidepressants often cause a dry mouth, but the complaint of dry mouth may also be a manifestation of depression;
- Tricyclic antidepressants interact with noradrenaline;
- Tricyclics and monoamine oxidase inhibitors (MAOI) do not significantly interact with adrenaline in dental local anaesthetic solutions;
- Tricyclics and fluoxetine are epileptogenic.

Agents for use in xerostomia (Table 10.11)

Referral to a specialist

Referral may be indicated when the practitioner is faced with:

- A possibly complicated or serious diagnosis (especially cancer, HIV infection, pemphigus);

Table 10.11   Some sialogogues and salivary replacements

Agent	Use	Comments
Sialogogues		
Pilocarpine (*Salagen*)	5 mg up to 3 times daily with food	Patient may be unable to see well enough to drive or operate machinery. Contraindicated in asthma, chronic obstructive airways disease, glaucoma, pregnancy. Care with cardiac disease
Salivix	Malic acid	Pastille
Salivary replacements (artificial salivas)	**Constituents**	
Glandosane	Sodium carboxymethylcellulose base	Spray
Luborant	Sodium carboxymethylcellulose base	Spray
Salivace	Sodium carboxymethylcellulose base	Spray
Saliveze	Sodium carboxymethylcellulose base	Spray
Oralbalance	Lactoperoxidase, glucose oxidase and xylitol	Gel
Saliva Orthana	Mucin	Spray containing fluoride, or lozenge. May be unsuitable if there are religious objections to porcine mucin.

- A doubtful diagnosis;
- A patient who has extra-oral lesions or possible systemic disease;
- Investigations required, but not possible, or appropriate to carry out, in general practice;
- A situation where therapy may not be straightforward and may require potent agents;
- A situation where drug use needs to be monitored with laboratory or other testing (for example for liver functional disturbances);

- A patient who needs access to an informed opinion outside normal working hours.

Should referral be required, it should always be in writing giving a concise background to the referral, including:

- Referring dental surgeon's name and address, telephone, facsimile and electronic mail;
- Patient's surname;
- Patient's first name(s);
- Patient's date of birth;
- Patient's full address and telephone, facsimile and electronic mail where possible;
- Patient's medical practitioner's name and address, telephone, facsimile and electronic mail;
- Urgency of referral;
- Reason for referral;
- Relevant history;
- Relevant findings;
- Provisional diagnosis;
- Relevant medical history;
- Treatment already offered.

Further reading

Allen CM. Diagnosing and managing oral candidiasis. *J Am Dent Assoc* (1992) **123**: 77.

Axell T et al. Evaluation of a simplified diagnostic aid (Oricult-N) for detection of oral candidoses. *Scand J Dent Res* (1985) **93**: 52.

Bagg J, Mannings A, Munro J, Walker DM. Rapid diagnosis of oral herpes simplex or zoster virus infections by immunofluorescence: comparison with Tzanck cell preparations and viral culture. *Br Dent J* (1989) **167**: 235–8.

Bedi R, Crawford AN. Assessment of the medical status of Asian immigrant children undergoing dental care. *J Dent* (1982) **10**: 144–8.

Bengel W. The ideal dental photographic system. *Quintessence Int* (1993) **24**: 251.

Brodell RT, Helms SE, Devine M. Office dermatologic testing: the Tzanck preparation. *Am Fam Physician* (1991) **44**: 857–60.

Chambers I, Scully C. Medical information from referral letters. *Oral Surg Oral Med Oral Pathol* (1987) **64**: 674–6.

Cohen PR. Tests for detecting herpes simplex virus and varicella-zoster virus infections. *Dermatol Clin* (1994) **12**: 51–68.

De Jong KJM, Abraham-Inpijn L, Oomen HAPC et al. Clinical relevance of a medical history in dental practice; comparison between a questionnaire and a dialogue. *Community Dent Oral Epidemiol* (1991) **19**: 310–1.

Dhariwal SK, Cubie HA, Southam JC. Detection of human papillomavirus in oral lesions using commercially developed typing kits. *Oral Microbiol Immunol* (1995) **10**: 60–3.

Dunne SM, Clark CG. The identification of the medically compromised patient in dental practice. *J Dent* (1985) **13**: 45–51.

Eisen D. The oral mucosal punch biopsy: a report of 140 cases. *Arch Dermatol* (1992) **128**: 815–17.

Epstein JB, Page JL, Anderson GH, Spinelli J. The role of an immunoperoxi-dase technique in the diagnosis of oral herpes simplex virus infection in patients with leukemia. *Diagn Cytopathol* (1987) **3**: 205–9.

Ficarra G, McClintock B, Hansen LS. Artifacts created during oral biopsy procedures. *J Craniomaxillofac Surg* (1987) **15**: 34–7.

Flaitz CM, Hammond HL. The immunoperoxidase method for the rapid diagnosis of intraoral herpes simplex virus infection in patients receiving bone marrow transplants. *Spec Care Dentist* (1988) **8**: 82–5.

Hampton JR, Harrison MJG, Mitchell JRA et al. Relative contributions of history-taking, physical examination and laboratory investigation to diagnosis and management of medical outpatients. *BMJ* (1975) **ii**: 486–9.

Harahap M. How to biopsy oral lesions. *J Dermatol Surg Oncol* (1989) **15**: 1077–80.

Jainkittivong A, Yeh C-K, Guest GF et al. Evaluation of medical consultations in a predoctoral dental clinic. *Oral Surg* (1995) **80**: 409–13.

Jones JH, Mason DK. *Oral Manifestations of Systemic Disease*, 2nd edn. (Baillière: London, 1980).

Kaplan EB, Sheiner LB, Boeckman AJ et al. The usefulness of preoperative laboratory screening. *J Am Med Assoc* (1985) **253**: 3576–81.

Lewis MAO, Samaranayake LP, Lamey PJ. Diagnosis and treatment of oral candidosis. *J Oral Maxillofac Surg* (1991) **49**: 996.

Luker J, Matthews R, Scully C. Radionuclide imaging in dentistry. *Postgrad Dent* (1993) **3**: 204–8.

Lynch DP, Gibson DK. The use of calcofluor white in the histopathologic diagnosis of oral candidiasis. *Oral Surg Oral Med Oral Pathol* (1987) **63**: 698–703.

Lynch DP, Morris LF. The oral mucosal punch biopsy: indications and technique. *J Am Dent Assoc* (1990) **121**: 145–9.

McDaniel TF, Miller D, Jones R et al. Assessing patient willingness to reveal health history information. *J Am Dent Assoc* (1995) **126**: 375–9.

MacPhail LA, Hilton JF, Heinic GS, Greenspan D. Direct immunofluorescence vs. culture for detecting HSV in oral ulcers: a comparison. *J Am Dent Assoc* (1995) **126**: 74–8.

Migliorati CA, Jones AC, Baughman PA. Use of exfoliative cytology in the diagnosis of oral hairy leukoplakia. *Oral Surg Oral Med Oral Pathol* (1993) **76**: 704–10.

Millard HD, Mason DK (eds). *Perspectives on 1993 World Workshop on Oral Medicine.* (University of Michigan: Ann Arbor, 1995).

Miller CS, Kaplan AL, Guest GF et al. Documenting medication use in adult dental patients; 1987–1991. *J Am Dent Assoc* (1992) **123**: 41–8.

Mintz GA, Rose SL. Diagnosis of oral herpes simplex virus infections: practical aspects of viral culture. *Oral Surg Oral Med Oral Pathol* (1984) **58**: 486–92.

Moenning JE, Tomich CE. A technique for fixation of oral mucosal lesions. *J Oral Maxillofac Surg* (1992) **50**: 1345.

Olsen L, Stenderup A. Clinical-mycologic diagnosis of oral yeast infections. *Acta Odontol Scand* (1990) **48**: 11–18.

Peacock ME, Carson RE. Frequency of self-reported medical conditions in periodontal patients. *J Periodontol* (1995) **66**: 1004–7.

Porter SR, Scully C, Welsby P, Gleeson M. *Colour Guide to Medicine and Surgery for Dentistry*, 2nd edn. (Churchill-Livingstone: Edinburgh, 1999).

Sciubba J. Improving detection of precancerous and cancerous oral lesions: computer-assisted analysis of oral brush biopsy. *JADA* (1999) **130**: 1445–57.

Scully C. Examination of the head and neck. Part I. *Student Update* (1980) **2**: 159.

Scully C. Examination of the head and neck. Part II. *Student Update* (1980) **2**: 197.

Scully C. Examination of the head and neck. Part III. *Student Update* (1980) **2**: 228.

Scully C. *Hospital Dental Surgeon's Guide*. (British Dental Journal: London, 1985).

Scully C. *The Dental Patient*. (Heinemann: Oxford, 1988).

Scully C. *The Mouth and Perioral Tissues*. (Heinemann: Oxford, 1989).

Scully C. *Patient Care: A Dental Surgeon's Guide*. (British Dental Journal: London, 1989).

Scully C. The new professional role of the dentist: internal medicine. In: *Interprofessional Cooperation in Dental Care*. (Institute der Deutschen Zahnarzte: Koln, 1993) 167–206.

Scully C. The new professional role of the dentist under aspects of internal medicine. *Int Dent J* (1993) **43**: 323–34.

Scully C. Diagnosis and diagnostic procedures: general and soft tissue diagnosis. In: *Pathways in Practice*. (Faculty of General Dental Practice, Royal College of Surgeons of England: London, 1993) 25–33.

Scully C. Inflammatory disorders of the oral mucosa. In: English GM, ed., *Otolaryngology*. (Lippincott: Philadelphia, 1993) 1–28.

Scully C. The pathology of orofacial disease. In: Barnes IE, Walls AWG, eds, *Gerodontology*. (Wright-Butterworths: Oxford, 1994) 29–41.

Scully C. Prevention of oral mucosal disease. In: Murray JJ, ed. *Prevention of oral and dental disease*. 3rd edn. (Oxford University Press: Oxford, 1995) 160–72.

Scully C, Boyle P. Reliability of a self-administered questionnaire for screening medical problems in dentistry. *Community Dent Oral Epidemiol* (1983) **11**: 105.

Scully C, Cawson RA. *Medical Problems in Dentistry*, 4th edn. (Wright: Bristol, 1998).

Scully C, Cawson RA. *Colour Guide To Oral Medicine*, 2nd edn. (Churchill-Livingstone: London, 1999).

Scully C. *Slide Interpretation in Oral Diseases*. (Oxford University Press: Oxford, 1999).

Sigvard P. Self-assessment of dental conditions: validity of a questionnaire. *Community Dent Oral Epidemiol* (1991) **19**: 249–51.

Skoglund A, Sunzel B, Lerner UH. Comparison of three test methods used for the diagnosis of candidiasis. *Scand J Dent Res* (1994) **102**: 295.

Sonis ST, Fazio R, Setkowicz A et al. Comparison of the nature and frequency of medical problems among patients in general speciality and hospital dental practices. *J Oral Med* (1983) **38**: 58–61.

Wagner JD, Moore DL. Preoperative laboratory testing for the oral and maxillofacial surgery patient. *J Oral Maxillofac Surg* (1991) **49**: 177–82.

Index

Granulomatous cheilitis, 200, 326–8
Granulomatous disease, chronic, 114
Graphite tattoos, 70, 72
Gustatory sweating, 42–3

Haemangiomas, 132–4
  senile of lip, 336–7
  Sturge–Weber syndrome, 223, 224
Haemorrhagic telangiectasia, 136–7
Hairy leukoplakia, 148, 149, 150,
    374–6
Hairy tongue, 360–2
Halitosis, 10–11
Hamartomas
  haemangiomas, 132–4
  lymphangioma, 179–80
  multiple, 114
Hand, foot and mouth disease,
    134–6
Hand–Schuller–Christian disease, 160
Hereditary angioneurotic oedema,
    309, 310
Hereditary benign intraepithelial
    dyskeratosis, 136
Hereditary gingival fibromatosis,
    288–9
Hereditary haemorrhagic
    telangiectasia, 136–7
Hereditary mucoepithelial dysplasia,
    137–8
Herpangina, 138–9, 342
Herpes simplex infections, 139–45,
    162, 163
  antiviral therapy, 400
  erythema multiforme, 321
  lips, 142–3, 163, 301, 328–30
  palate, 143, 144, 342
Herpes zoster (shingles), 43–5, 109,
    236–8, 400
Herpetic neuralgia, 43–5
Herpetic stomatitis, primary, 140–2,
    144, 145
Herpetiform ulcers, 78, 80–1
Hexetidine, 391
Histiocytosis X *see* Langerhans' cell
    histiocytoses
Histology specimens, 389
Histopathological terms, 67

Histoplasmosis, 145–6
History taking, 385
Hodgkin's lymphoma, 181, 183
Human immunodeficiency virus
    infection, 146–51, 153, 159
  drug therapy, 396
  Kaposi's sarcoma, 150
  lymphomas, 181, 182, 183
  tuberculosis, 228, 229
  warts, 232
  see also AIDS patients
Human papillomaviruses, 159, 202,
    232
Hydrocortisone, 82, 394
Hydroxychloroquine, 397
Hygiene, oral, 390, 391
Hyperkeratosis, definition, 67
Hyperparathyroidism, 286, 287
Hyperpigmentation, 12–13, 68–70,
    123, 192–5, 303
Hyperplasia
  adenomatoid, 344
  drug-induced gingival, 283–5
  papillary, 351
  pseudocarcinomatous, 67, 214
Hyperplastic candidiasis, 98, 99,
    157–9
Hyperplastic gingivitis, 280
Hypoaesthesia, 1, 2

Idiopathic circumorificial
    plasmacytosis, 295
Idiopathic trigeminal neuralgia, 46,
    49–51
IgA deficiency, 114
IgA disease, linear, 175–6, 396
Immunocompromised patients
  antifungal agents, 397, 400
  candidiasis, 94, 95, 98, 99–100
  herpes simplex infections, 143,
    145, 329, 330
  histoplasmosis, 146
  Kaposi's sarcoma, 349
  leukaemia, 161–3
  lymphoma, 181–3
  organ transplants, 226–7
  rhinocerebral zygomycosis, 190
  shingles, 236, 237